Explaining the Brain

Explaining the Brain

W. RITCHIE RUSSELL

with
A. J. DEWAR
(M.R.C. Brain Metabolism Unit, Edinburgh)

OXFORD UNIVERSITY PRESS

Oxford University Press, Walton Street, Oxford

OXFORD LONDON GLASGOW NEW YORK TORONTO MELBOURNE
WELLINGTON CAPE TOWN IBADAN NAIROBI DAR ES SALAAM LUSAKA
DELHI BOMBAY CALCUTTA MADRAS KARACHI KUALA LUMPUR
SINGAPORE JAKARTA HONG KONG TOKYO

ISBN 0 19 289079 4

© OXFORD UNIVERSITY PRESS 1975

First published 1975
Reprinted 1977

Printed in Great Britain by
Fletcher & Son Ltd
Norwich

Preface

Our brains are very special, for the development of the human brain is apparently the key to man's superiority over other animals.

It seems probable that, during evolution, man's brain enlarged as he acquired hand-skills. This gave him an enormous advantage over all other species, and in the process of natural selection within the human species must have come to act in favour of those possessing better hand-skills. The development of these hand-skills presumably preceded man's capacity for speech, which in turn led to the development of increasingly complex thinking and reasoning, and ultimately to man's using his brain in the way that we all do today.

Healthy human brains at birth are all much alike, so that each intact human being is born with an astonishingly intricate package that provides capacity for achievement or failure, pleasure or unhappiness, genius or nonentity. The genetic codes transmitted by the father and mother determine the detailed structure of the body; but although ten thousand million nerve cells are present at birth, the connections between them are laid down afterwards—during the early months and years of life—and the effectiveness with which they come to intercommunicate must depend chiefly, if not entirely, on early environmental factors. It is therefore vital that we should all have a simple working knowledge of how to use and take care of our brains and those of the infants who may be in our care, so that we may provide environments in which healthy, active brains may mature.

It is imperative that a child should be adequately stimulated if his brain is to develop its full potential, and I shall return to this theme repeatedly throughout this book. However, it is just as vital that the child should be given every chance of reasonable brain development before birth. This depends, of course, on maintaining the health of the mother at a high level through pregnancy—a fact which should not be ignored when considering the happiness and welfare of our next generation. We should all now be wary of administering to the mother such brain-active drugs as thalidomide—or even achohol, nicotine, and barbiturates —which will have a far greater effect on her unborn infant than on herself. The alarming fact is that, although the mature adult's brain can be severely damaged without much change in capacity, a similar injury to the foetal brain is likely to reduce future potential to perhaps a small fraction of what could otherwise have been expected.

During later life our brains may be at risk from disease, malnutrition, head injury, or from commonly used drugs, and, in order to see these matters in reasonable perspective, we should all know something of how the brain works.

Because the brain is so complex it is extremely difficult to find out how it works, or even how a small section works; unless something goes wrong. When we discover that a particular sort of injury produces a specific disability (say inability to read) we learn a little about how the healthy brain must have been coping with the problem of reading. This is why we learn so much from the study of brain injuries, and why so much of this book is concerned with them—not because most brains are damaged, but because our best understanding of the working of the brain comes from seeing what happens when something goes wrong.

Against this somewhat harsh background of current knowledge many will also find it useful to study the relationship between the brain and the mind. In past centuries man could conclude only that his brain, mind, and soul must be quite separate entities—indeed the role of the brain in generating a 'mind' or 'soul' was not even thought about.

Throughout the ages, one of man's most cherished beliefs has always been that he has a separate soul. The evidence in support of this traditional belief has become unconvincing in the light of modern knowledge, and in order to avoid ambiguity in this book, I have written with the assumption that man has neither a soul nor a spirit.

Nowadays the word 'mind' is used as a convenient term for describing what we loosely refer to as the 'thinking aspects' of brain activity. I myself find it most rational to think on these lines, so that when referring to the mind, I intend to convey a picture of certain patterns of brain activity. In this book I suggest that some people have two minds; this argument is analogous to the psychologist's reference to people having two personalities, but with the additional physiological concept that two minds operate through differing groups of 'electrical' circuits within the same brain. The exact choice of terminology is not important, but the idea is a useful one when describing the reactions of people with hysterical personalities or the rather similar responses seen from the effects of hypnosis (see Chapter 4).

I hope that the reader of these pages will feel he is helped by acquiring some knowledge of his brain. It may be too late to change our own brain very much, but we can learn to enjoy cultivating what we have, and what is more important, can learn more effectively how to help later generations.

W.R.R.

Oxford, 1975

Contents

Chapters 9 and 10 were written in conjunction with Dr. A. J. Dewar, of
the Medical Research Council Brain Metabolism Unit, and are based
largely on his special knowledge and experience.

I

What is a brain?

When we meet a close acquaintance in the street, we use a routine of which we may be hardly aware. Let us consider what happens.

1. We expect to recognize the face.
2. We expect to remember the name.
3. We have complete confidence that our correlation of name and face is correct.
4. We remember our past associations with this acquaintance, and our welcome is adjusted accordingly.
5. We make an appropriate verbal comment, or other signs of recognition.
6. We experience pleasure, or the reverse, at the meeting.
7. When we part, we can remember the meeting, at least for a day or two.
8. Should the meeting prove to be extremely significant we may remember it for the rest of our lives, or for as long as our brains are healthy—whichever is the shorter.

For each of these hardly considered actions and emotions different areas of the brain must be involved in activating millions of nerve cells to produce the expected response, and at the same time millions of other nerve cells must be temporarily blocked in order not to confuse the mechanism. This is a highly efficient 'silent service' which we all take for granted until one or more parts of the mechanism begins to fail as a result of neglect, misuse, disease, or old age. Then we notice what we have lost for ever.

In this chapter, I shall endeavour to describe the construction of the complex system which supports us in every action and thought throughout our lives. This system is known as the central nervous system, and consists of the brain and the spinal cord (see Fig. 1).

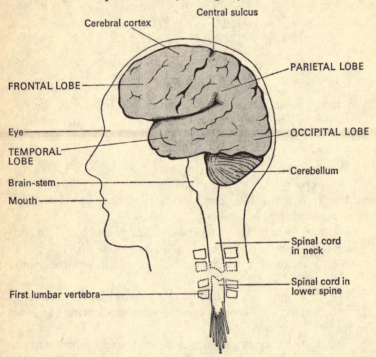

FIG. 1. Diagram to illustrate the position of the brain and spinal cord in the human head and spine.

The brain receives information from the sense organs and all parts of the body, via the nerves and spinal cord. It analyses this input in the light of its memory of past experiences, and has final control over any purposeful reaction to the information received. The transmission system to and from the brain, and also the analysis within the brain, are dependent on a vast number of nerve cells (neurones)—every healthy human infant is born with about ten thousand million of them.

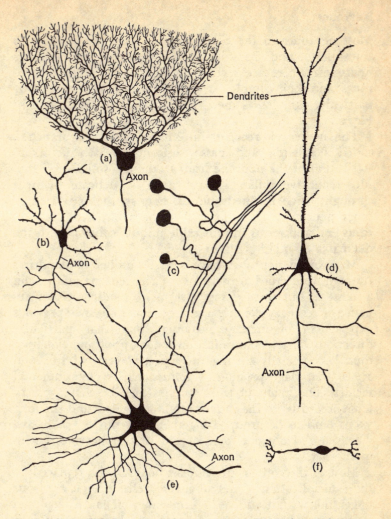

FIG. 2. Some different types of neurone: (a) From the cerebellum—
note the elaborate branching of the dendrites; (b) Brain cell with a
short axon; (c) Spinal ganglion cells; (d) Cell from the motor cortex
of the brain with a long axon on its way to the spinal cord; (e) Motor
cell from the spinal cord with a long axon on its way to a muscle;
(f) Nerve cell from the retina.

Neurones

Most neurones in the brain seem to have the capacity to transmit to, and share in, the activation of several other neurones. There are several different kinds of these neurones, and their complex structure varies according to their particular function; some of the varieties are illustrated in Fig. 2.

The nerve cell receives information from its branches, called dendrites, and passes information via its axon. Activation of the neurone leads to the transmission of rapidly repetitive pulses via the axon—a delicate filament through which the neurone can help in the activation of other neurones. To achieve this, the axon branches near to its end and forms innumerable minute contacts with the dendrites of other neurones.

Most brain neurones have a vast number of dendrites through which they are activated. Each neurone can pass on a message, but in so doing it seems to modify—either enhance or reduce—the message, according to its own previous experiences of messages coming from that particular direction. These communication systems grow and elaborate quickly, especially during the first two years of life, and are at that stage profoundly influenced by environmental factors. The axons of the neurones may be short or very long, according to the distance to be travelled, and the long axons tend to be grouped together in bands or 'pathways' which lead from one part of the central nervous system to another.

Most of the cells in the human body can be replaced by the multiplication of neighbouring cells: if you cut your finger the wound will heal; skin flakes off and is replaced continuously; even fractured bones will knit together in a few weeks. We are not able to grow new limbs or new organs, but self-repair on a small scale is efficient. However, brain cells are quite different, and if a brain neurone dies it can never be replaced.

The double brain

The brains of all animals show close similarities of structure, and the size and complexity of the brain seems to determine the status of the species in the animal kingdom. In most species the central nervous system is divided into two halves—right and left—which seem to be identical to each

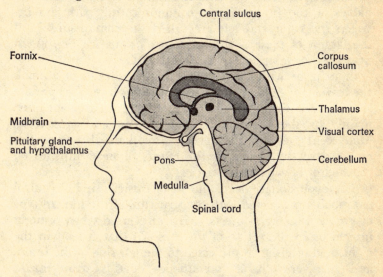

Fig. 3. The left half of the brain (the left cerebral hemisphere) has been cut away by dividing the commissures (darker in the diagram). In this way the inside of the right cerebral hemisphere has been exposed, and the double nature of the structure can be seen. In the brain-stem (pons and medulla), the right and left halves are fused together as they are in the spinal cord, but the cerebral hemispheres are well separated except where they communicate with each other via the commissures.

other in structure and size. These two halves are well separated from each other in, say, the nervous system of a worm, but in more advanced animals the right and left halves are fused together within the spinal cord and brain. In the brain, these two halves are called the cerebral hemispheres. This structure is often referred to as a double brain, and has some unique features in man.

Most animals have a leading-end, where the eyes and the brain have evolved. In an environment that is dominated by the force of gravity, the development of the double central nervous system is a method of solving the problem of preserving stability during movement. It is not surprising therefore, to find that in all animals there is extensive and elaborate provision for communication between the two halves of the brain. These communicating pathways between the right and left are called the commissures, and the largest of these is the corpus callosum (see Fig. 3). In man they are extremely well developed.

In man, as with many of the higher species of animal, the main control of one side of the body is from the opposite side of the brain. Thus, the right arm and leg are controlled mainly by the left cerebral hemisphere, and vice versa. Many centuries ago, the ancient Egyptians discovered this cross-control by observing the effects of head injuries on the bodies of wounded warriors.

The evolutionary development of this crossing of control is probably connected with the structure of the human type of eye, in which all objects seen are reversed when brought into focus in the retina of the eye. All that is seen in the right field of vision is projected to the left side of the brain, and vice versa. As a consequence of this arrangement, danger seen from the right and movement-control of the right arm are both effected from the same side of the brain (the left). This is an obvious advantage.

A leading cerebral hemisphere

For many purposes, the right and left cerebral hemispheres seem to operate in unison. For example, basic decisions on which survival depends, such as whether to run away from danger, seem to become habitual as a result of innumerable past experiences, and these may become almost as automatic as is the knowledge of how to walk or to run. Some animals bred in captivity fail to develop the self-preservation reactions required for life in the wild, presumably through lack of relevant experience.

In contrast to these relatively primitive forms of choice, for which both halves of the brain seem to work as one, man's more complex types of choice and decision are associated with a unique concentration of certain skills in either one or other of the cerebral hemispheres. The most important of these special developments is that the *left* cerebral hemisphere usually dominates man's language skills. Man is far better than all other species at communicating by speech, and in addition he can be taught both to read and to write. The term 'aphasia' (see p. 59) is used to include any disturbances of the speech mechanism which result from brain disease or injury.

Brain-damaged victims of the Second World War provided invaluable information about the speech mechanisms of the brain. Most of the non-fatal brain wounds were caused by small fragments of metal which travelled at high velocity and destroyed very localized areas of the brain. Aphasia appeared in only three per cent of the cases injured in the *right* cerebral hemisphere, but in victims damaged in the *left* cerebral hemisphere, aphasia followed in sixty per cent of the cases. Furthermore, in these latter cases wounds in the left frontal lobes rarely led to speech disturbances, but wounds above the left ear (left parietal lobe —see Fig. 1) nearly always caused aphasia and paralysis of the right hand.

Right-handed or left-handed?

Another unique feature in man is the frequency with which one or other side of the brain is specially connected with motor skills, particularly the delicate control of muscular activity required for hand-skills. Again the left cerebral hemisphere is usually dominant. This arrangement is usually associated with right-handedness, and of course most people are right-handed. About eighty per cent of the population are right-handed, ten per cent left-handed, and ten per cent ambidextrous.

There has been a natural tendency to assume that in a right-handed person the left cerebral hemisphere is also dominant for language, and in a left-handed person the right hemisphere is dominant for language, but this correlation is by no means constant. Some left-handers use the left side of the brain for language, and a few right-handers use the right side of the brain for language.

Here it should be made clear that a dominant side exerting its control over language or hand-skills operates via both sides of the brain, so that in speaking both vocal cords and both sides of the tongue, face, and throat act together. Similarly, information from the ears and eyes comes to both sides of the brain but is passed to the dominant side for special language analysis. This specialist concentration in the dominant language hemisphere is largely acquired soon after birth. Thus an adult who experiences severe destruction of the dominant hemisphere by disease or injury will never completely recover from the aphasia, whereas a child of two or three years of age who experiences a similar injury is able to switch the development of his language mechanism to what was otherwise developing as the non-dominant or 'minor' hemisphere. In other words, the development of one side of the brain for special skills must involve the formation of special physical changes in communication between neurones, which cannot be replaced by similar changes in the other side of the brain after growth to maturity. This most important aspect of the learning mechanisms will be considered further in the next chapter.

There is now evidence that it is not only for language functions and motor skills that man's brain concentrates its resources on one side; it seems that many people use the minor hemisphere (usually the *right* side of the brain) for such skills as visual pattern recognition.

We do not know why the left side of the brain should usually be used for language and hand-skills. Both of these groups of skills start to be developed at an early age, and I think that the reason might be very simple. Perhaps the left side of the brain usually matures earlier during infancy because there is a slightly better blood-supply to that side at birth. Certainly the left hemisphere acquires its dominance during the first four or five years of life.

The specialization of hemispheres may well be connected in some way with man's unique potential for learning. It is tempting to suggest that the processes involved are so complex, and involve so many millions of the brain cells, that duplication on both sides would not only be very wasteful but might become incompatible with sanity.

Whether the so-called 'mind' operates more in one hemisphere than the other is not at all clear. Indeed some people seem to have more than one mind, a theme to which I shall return later.

2

The development and degeneration of brain and mind

In man, the nervous system is well developed at birth. Most of the ten thousand million neurones have already been formed, and most are positioned approximately where they will remain for as long as they survive. Even at birth these neurones have crude connections with at least some other neurones and, as maturity progresses, they learn to co-operate with increasing efficiency. The vast majority of the central nervous system neurones are in the cerebral hemispheres, but there are many nerve cells in every section of the brain-stem and spinal cord. For example, the spinal cord contains about ten thousand brain cells that activate movement for each limb of the body. These 'motor' cells are the nerve cells whose axons directly activate the muscles of the arms and legs. They are destroyed, for example, in polio (paralytic poliomyelitis), a disease caused by a virus that attacks the nervous system.

Regeneration of nerves

The motor tracts, consisting of axons from motor cells, pass down the brain-stem and spinal cord to activate the dendrites of the spinal-cord motor cells. From here, the axons of the spinal-cord motor cells extend from the spinal cord to the muscles they supply in, say, the hand or the leg. These long axons leave the spinal cord via the spinal 'nerve roots', and then become rearranged to be incorporated in the nerves going to the various muscles of the limbs and body. The spinal-cord motor cells (motor neurones) are irreplaceable after destruction (as in poliomyelitis), but if a nerve in, say, the arm is crushed or divided, the motor axons will grow down again (regenerate) if the cut ends of the nerve are sewn together. This process is often imperfect, and takes place over a period of many months.

Unfortunately the regenerating axons may branch and go to the wrong muscle, or to more than one muscle, and such regeneration results in an imperfect recovery of function. This is commonly seen in those who have at one time had one side of the face paralysed by a nerve injury or neuritis (Bell's palsy) which has required regeneration for recovery. In these instances the movements of the one side of the face are always somewhat distorted, as the muscles on that side tend to contract together, so that, for example, a blink of the eyelids may be accompanied by a slight twitch of that side of the mouth, and a smile may always cause a slight eyelid movement resembling a wink. On one occasion I recognized this anomaly in a middle-aged man who told me that the previous facial paralysis had been caused at his birth by the use of forceps!

Transmission of impulses between neurones

As already described, each neurone in the brain develops outgrowths through which it is in contact with other nerve cells or with sense organs. Fig. 2 (p. 3) illustrates the dendrites which feed into the cell body from 'up-stream', and the axon which transmits 'down-stream' impulses from the cell to other neurones. Some axons are very short; but when it joins the large tracts a single axon may stretch from the brain to the lower spine. As the nerve-cell body is barely visible to the naked eye (it is about 0.04 mm in diameter) the axon may stretch for a distance that is over thirty thousand times the width of the cell from which it grows. If all the axons and dendrites from one brain could be added end to end to form a wire, this wire would be long enough to encircle the Earth several times.

An electrical current will activate an axon to transmit

an impulse throughout its length, but the pulse in nerves is by no means a purely electrical phenomenon for it travels at a rate of only about forty metres a second (ten million times more slowly than electricity). The strength of the message sent down the axon seems to depend on the frequency of the pulses rather than the strengths of the individual pulses. The frequency of the pulses can rise to over 400 a second, so that individual pulses following each other down a long tract may be only about ten centimetres apart.

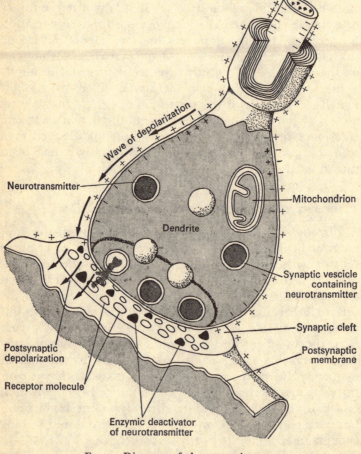

FIG. 4. Diagram of the synaptic gap.

The communicating systems between one neurone and another are called 'synapses' (Fig. 4). These are very complex and are formed by the axons of up-stream neurones meeting the dendrites of the receiving cell. The axons and dendrites involved do not touch but are separated by a small gap (the 'synaptic cleft') across which activation is passed from one neurone to the next. This process of transmission is effected by the liberation of a chemical (called a 'neurotransmitter') which will be discussed further in Chapter 9.

The differing types of neurone are grouped in special areas within the brain, but are rather vaguely classified—one particular criterion being that the different types of neurone often have differing chemical mechanisms, using different chemicals as neurotransmitters (see Chapter 9). These differences are of great practical importance, for they enable us to understand partly the reason why certain chemicals or drugs apparently act on only one type of neurone. The drug *curare* completely paralyses the limb and body muscles (by blocking the transmission of impulses from axon to muscle) without disturbing consciousness or reducing the appreciation of pain. Some drugs cause sleep without paralysis, and others cause visions (hallucinations) which seem to be due to false activation of the delicate recalling and memory systems. There have been important discoveries about drugs that act on one facet of the central nervous system activity, which have recently led to some significant advances in medical treatment of disease or malfunction of the brain. We shall discuss psychoactive drugs of this variety in Chapter 9.

A neurone does much more than merely transmit pulses from one cell to another, for it also has the ability to change the strength of its responses to incoming stimuli, and thus to modulate the impulse it transmits. This continual readjustment of the neurones seems to be most active during the years of maturation, and these responses must be closely connected with the physiology of learning. After maturity is reached learning ability deteriorates but continues to some extent as long as the brain is healthy (but see p. 104).

The eventual outcome of the neurone's adjustment to the influence from other neurones is probably determined by a simple quantitative effect (like any good democratic process). The most frequently used pathway from other cells is strengthened and preserved and may eventually become so well established that a tiny but firm link is formed in what will become the chain of a life-long habit. For example, by the time maturity is reached, a man has developed a characteristic habit of posture and movement, and his signature is so fixed as to be honoured by his bank.

The neuronal reactions involved in language, thought, and intellectual types of activity are so complex that they may always remain beyond human comprehension. On the other hand, the capacity of the brain is so immense that I think it is reasonable to consider that the behaviour of an *individual* neurone of a particular variety may well be the same whatever its sphere of activity. It is not the individual activity but the vast numbers of neurones involved that becomes impossible to grasp. Little wonder that the research worker keeps turning to study the individual neurone, which seems to possess such remarkable versatility.

Neurones have an unusually high metabolic rate, that is, they 'live faster' than most cells (metabolism is explained in Chapter 9). The process of metabolism continues without ceasing by day and night, and it is tempting to speculate that most of this activity is concerned not only with the elemental task of transmission but also with the complex business of consolidating the most important changes caused by the experience of recent bombardment via the dendrites.

Enemies of the neurone

Owing partly to their very high metabolic rate, neurones are vulnerable to a lack of oxygen, which may be caused by an insufficiency of the blood circulation; and of course if they are destroyed they can never be replaced. Neurones are also destroyed in large numbers by concussion, by strokes (caused by blockage of a brain artery), by heat stroke, by encephalitis (inflammation of the brain), and probably also by severe exhaustion, which can disrupt the circulation to the brain when the subject is in an erect posture.

It is quite likely that people who go to all-night parties after a day's work run a considerable risk of losing many brain cells. Many drugs are also known to disturb the control of circulation when the taker is in the upright position, and the not uncommon habit of going to sleep sitting up in a corner of a room while both exhausted and under the influence of drugs must be particularly dangerous.

Some experts believe that, even without any of these unusual stresses, brain cells begin to disappear by the age of about twenty at a rate of thousands every day.

During growth and development man, like all animals, is engaged in a struggle for existence with the many potential enemies in his environment. These include other animals, micro-organisms, viruses, man-made chemicals, and some products of the vegetable kingdom. Animals require a safe and balanced diet, but many chemicals are toxic—for example the brain is particularly vulnerable to mercury poisoning. On the other hand, a trace of many elements is necessary for survival—for example, a lack of copper in the soil leads to a fatal interference with brain growth in sheep (the disease 'swayback').

Another important example of the nutritional needs of the brain is the special vulnerability of a certain system of the brain (the limbic system; see p. 96) to a lack of vitamin B (which is found in bread, meat, oatmeal, and soya products). This vitamin deficiency may lead to destruction of an essential part of this system, as occurs in alcoholic insanity (Wernicke's encephalopathy), in which a rapidly developing and irrecoverable mental failure takes place unless corrective treatment is provided early in the illness.

The vast number of chemicals produced by plants include some that have a powerful influence on the animal brain. In the course of plant evolution, it is obvious that any plant which has managed to develop chemicals poisonous to animals, insects, or viruses has provided a wonderful boost towards the survival of its particular species, and likewise animal species which avoid poisonous plants are most likely to survive. To give a homely example, the seedlings of foxglove and nicotina (containing digitalis and nicotine) seem to be shunned by snails.

Most herbs that are used in cooking or are used therapeutically in man are poisonous to some insects that would otherwise eat them, but as yet insufficient research has been done on this interesting problem. Nowadays man-made chemicals are subject to strict scrutiny and research before being released for use, especially since the disasters caused by the use of thalidomide drugs. Incidentally, it is doubtful whether the dangers of thalidomide would yet have been discovered had the drug not been used on a vast scale—a disturbing thought. But many of the therapeutically used herbs have never been carefully scrutinized from this point of view. Who knows how many brain-cell killers or potential 'thalidomides' may lurk unseen in our medicine cabinets or in our collection of herbs for cooking?

Development of the brain in early life

During intra-uterine life, the brain neurones are already engaged in connecting up with the spinal cord and muscles, which is why the foetus is so active. After birth, the central nervous system begins its life-long battle with the environment. At first its activity seems to be concerned with the formation of purposeful movements of limbs, head, and eyes. This process involves endless repetitions which are constantly modified, leading to improvement. This struggle to improve performance continues until maturity, by which time highly skilled movements should have been learned.

The adjustments of the neurones that take place in relation to the processes of learning are as yet little understood, but considerable time is required to establish a 'memory trace' and it seems likely that a vast number of repetitions of the necessary patterns of impulses between neurones are required for the pattern to be retained (that is, learned).

At birth, though most of the neurones are in their proper place within the central nervous system, the connections of their axons and dendrites are poorly formed, but these develop greatly during the first two years of life. It seems very likely therefore that the very earliest environmental influences have a fundamental effect on the structure of interneuronal connections on which future activities depend.

Although there must be an enormous element of chance affecting the influences which determine these early structural patterns, let us approach the problem from the opposite direction by considering the exceptional skills of, for example, talented musicians. It is probably inconceivable that any great musician could have developed his talents unless he had been exposed to music in a pleasurable and personal way almost from the day of his birth. Without this very early and continued musical experience, the special elaboration of the hearing areas in his brain would not occur. I would suggest that young children who on reaching school age are found to be 'tone deaf', or unable to sing in tune, may have been deprived of suitable experience of music, and especially of singing, during the early months of life. There can be little doubt that many other special skills can develop only if that part of the brain most needed is used actively in the early months of life.

I have described how it seems very likely that the early uses of brain mechanisms have a profound influence on *structural* development in the brain; if this is so, many aspects of current educational practice must be reconsidered. For example, the elimination of illiteracy in healthy children seems to be a desirable object which could be achieved by familiarizing children with symbols from a very early age. This subject is considered in more detail in Chapter 11.

There is other and more basic evidence about this need to use a function of the brain if it is to develop. If a child is born with two perfect eyes, except that one is slightly long-sighted, the child comes to use the better eye alone and to ignore the slightly blurred view from the second-best eye; as the 'lazy' eye is not used for fixation, a slight squint develops. If the parents and doctor recognize this situation at a very early age and make the child wear glasses, the sight in the lazy eye will develop normally, but if the error is not corrected the lazy eye will quickly become permanently incapable of ever acquiring good vision, even if correct glasses are subsequently prescribed, and even if by some accident the sight of the good eye is lost. The lazy eye can never recover because it was not used during the first few years of life. From the structural point of view the retina of the eye is a part of the brain, and there are good reasons for concluding that vigorous activity by all parts of the brain is desirable from the earliest months of life if efficient development of the potential is to be achieved. This really amounts to a physiological fact, and makes nonsense of some current theories about the ways in which the environment of young children should be planned.

At the present, early brain development is providing a very active research field, and many studies are being made on environmental influences affecting the development of newly born animals. Some of the results are quite startling, and firmly support the view that the first months of life are extremely important in relation to future potential.

The mind

In the chapters that follow I have attempted to describe some of the methods by which information coming into the brain (especially via the eyes) is processed to the individual's best advantage, and the unique methods whereby man can use language to clarify his thought processes and to assist him in making better decisions. All these matters are fairly well understood, but we still have much to learn about what we usually term our 'minds'.

In order to try and appreciate the structure of what we call the mind, it may be helpful to study the thoughts and conversation of an elderly relative who is becoming some-what forgetful, for the highly repetitive responses will disclose the framework of patterns around which life-long activities and attitudes have been built. As we all know, the same remark repeated at varying intervals is likely to lead to exactly the same answer, the same story, or the same discourse, clearly demonstrating the enormous strength and rigidity of early patterns of activity.

Much of life involves the making of decisions to carry out activities of one kind or another, and people vary greatly in their ability to 'make up their minds'. It now seems to me that many people have at least two minds, and this causes both confusion and difficulty when considering the 'power of mind over matter' (which is discussed further on p. 36). This concept raises many questions.

Nowadays it is common practice to bring up children partly to believe in a happy fantasy-world and partly in an atmosphere that is uncomfortably realistic. Does this common practice encourage a life of two minds, and if so, is such an arrangement helpful or harmful? Many children in our Western civilisation are encouraged to believe in magic, miracles, fairies, spooks, and legendary creatures. Most of these beliefs and fantasies are probably harmless and often comforting to escape to when life is unhappy, and they may also provide the grounding necessary for creating the adult ability to 'escape' from the harsh realities of life.

Where people do seem to develop two separate minds, does mind A really know what mind B is thinking about?— or do the two minds become isolated from each other as might occur, for example, in a hysterical trance or under the effect of hypnotism? The question is far from simple to answer, although in the case of major 'hysterical' (psychosomatic) phenomena (causing apparent coma, blindness, fits, paralysis, and so on) mind A may have decided to 'hand over' to mind B in order to escape from an intolerable situation (see Chapter 4).

Despite the difficulties in defining what we mean by the human mind, some of which have been touched on in the preceding paragraphs, there seems to be no logical difficulty in considering man's mind to be a reflection of the activity of the brain, and this is how I shall regard it in the following chapters.

3

How the central nervous system works

The supremacy of man depends on the excess development of his brain compared with other species, and in particular on the great spread of the cortex of the cerebral hemispheres.

The cortex

The cortex covers the cerebral hemispheres with a blanket consisting of hundreds of millions of neurones which lie in several layers over most cortical areas. Each of these six or seven layers is distinguished from the others by being made up of a particular size and shape of nerve cell, although the significance of this arrangement is little understood. These outside layers of cortical cells are what we commonly refer to as 'grey matter' (see Fig. 5).

The 'white matter' of the brain lies within this blanket of grey matter and is made up mainly of long and short nerve-cell fibres, which carry impulses on their journeys through the brain. Like all nerve cells, the neurones of the cortex have complex communications not only with one another, but also with other important centres of the central nervous system. For example, it is known that a great flow of nerve fibres, particularly from the thalamus (see Fig. 6), arrives in the cortex to communicate with layer 4 of the cortical cells, while the great down-going tracts from cortex to spinal cord and brain-stem are formed from the axons of the large cells in layer 5. Indeed, layer 5 seems to provide the main means of communication from any part of the cortex to another part of the brain.

The control of instinctive behaviour

The cortex is not a separate entity, but an outgrowth or elaboration of the whole collection of more elementary brain mechanisms, and it maintains important and active communication systems with the brain-stem and spinal cord.

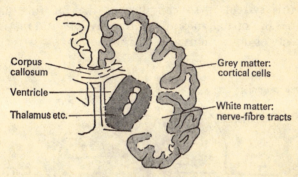

Corpus callosum

Ventricle

Thalamus etc.

Grey matter: cortical cells

White matter: nerve-fibre tracts

FIG. 5. A transverse vertical section of one cerebral hemisphere. The 'grey matter' forms a mantle or blanket over the whole surface of the brain and its surface is greatly increased by repeated infolding of the surface. Within this mantle lie the cortical neurones in their hundreds of millions, making the mantle appear relatively dark in colour to the naked eye. The 'white matter' appears to the naked eye to be relatively white in colour. This white matter consists mainly of short and long tracts of nerve-cell fibres (axons) conveying impulses from one part of the brain to another, including the thalamus and other nerve-cell centres deep in the brain, and of course to the other side of the brain via the corpus callosum. Another reason for the grey matter being darker in colour is that there are many more blood-vessels among nerve cells than among the fibres which form the white matter. This difference is more evident in adult life than in infancy.

In all animals it seems that the basic behavioural responses are moulded by a mechanism through which the advantageous is encouraged while what is harmful is discouraged or avoided. This mechanism is vital for survival. It controls the instinct to run away from danger, or the decision that it would be more advantageous to stay and fight. It also directs the emotional responses which we refer to as pleasure, anger, love, or hate.

These responses depend on the memory of the effects of all previous similar experiences. It is not surprising therefore to find that all these 'feeling' responses (including sexual responses) as well as the vital processes of memory, require that the brain-stem structures be intact. In man, these brain-stem mechanisms are closely connected with, and elaborated by, vast areas of cortex in the frontal lobes, and this system is so complicated that at this stage it becomes impossible to pinpoint the physiological motivation for many of our actions and decisions.

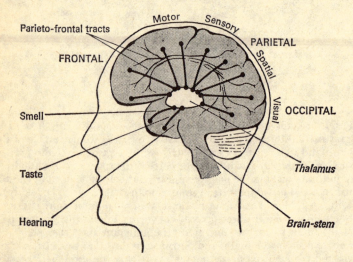

FIG. 6. The cerebral cortex is connected primarily with the thalamus, which lies in the middle of the hemisphere, and in this diagram the close intercommunications between cortex and thalamus are shown —apparently the cortex can do little or nothing without support from the thalamus. There is also a direct communication system between the parietal regions and the frontal lobes; this must be of great significance in relation to the transfer of current experience to the thought mechanism.

Alerting: the 'what-is-it?' mechanism

The brain-stem controlling systems (Fig. 7) also exert a most important function by alerting the brain to any unusual

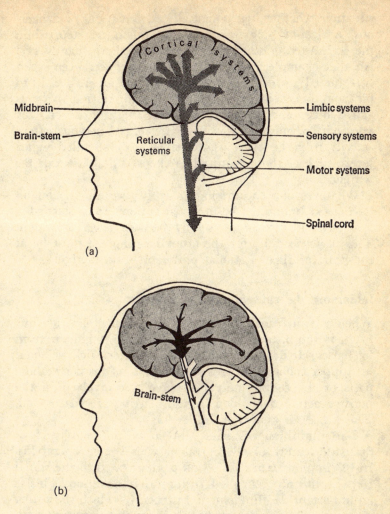

FIG. 7. The brain works day and night, but it only pays attention to the environment when alerted to do so. This phenomenon of being alerted is effected by a slender but powerful pathway to all parts of the brain and spinal cord which originates in cells in the brain-stem (the reticular system); this must be a primitive reflex for survival. (a) Illustrates this process of alerting, although the process is probably usually initiated from the opposite direction—from the parietal lobes to the brain-stem. (b) There are also corresponding inhibitory mechanisms which have the opposite effect.

situation, whether it is potentially advantageous or danger-ous. A sleeping dog wakens to an unfamiliar step, while the exhausted mother wakens only to her infant's cry. Another example is the 'cocktail party' effect: even when surrounded by many people talking, we are still able to pick out one voice saying something interesting, perhaps at the other end of the room. This amazing capacity for selectivity permeates all levels of the central nervous system activity, from the levels just described to the so-called higher levels, such as those required to choose suitable words for sentences.

Whatever our backgrounds may be, we all depend on having our brains alerted to pay attention—to be startled—or to have our interest aroused by the 'what-is-it?' activation. This basic necessity for the arousal of interest must be at the heart of all educational philosophy and method.

Inhibition: the concentration mechanism

When a man reads a newspaper or watches television, his brain is inhibiting many of the stimuli reaching it from his senses. He does not actively hear the clock ticking, smell his supper cooking, or 'feel' all the parts of his body; those parts of the central nervous system not involved in the positive action demanded by the alerting are inactivated. This process is known as 'inhibition'.

The inhibition of 'irrelevant' nerve-cell activity is a dramatic feature of all central nervous system operations. In its simplest form this is well demonstrated in the spinal cord by the process called reciprocal innervation. This is an important and fundamental process by which the strong contraction of one muscle group is usually associated with relaxation of the opposing muscles—the antagonists. For example, the contraction of the muscles of breathing is controlled by nerve cells in the brain-stem and in the spinal cord. Whilst breathing in, the muscles used for breathing out relax, and vice versa. This important inhibiting mech-anism is known to operate directly on the nerve cells which control the muscles from the spinal cord, and it seems

likely that this elementary example of inhibition is very
similar to the enormous number of processes of inhibition
which permeate all aspects of central nervous system
activity.

We are inclined to assume that the decision to, say, throw
a ball, actively provokes the arm area in the brain to repeat
a well-learned pattern of positive action. On the other hand,
the natural urge of motor cells to act is so powerful that
some experts think it more likely that the action is provided
by a carefully controlled pattern of releasing the constant
inhibition to which all motor cells must be submitted.

A frightening and dangerous example of the importance of
inhibition is seen in the muscle spasms of strychnine poisoning or of the disease tetanus ('lock-jaw'). It is now known
that these fearful spasms are not due to any form of irritation
or over-action of the motor nerve cells, but result from the
inhibitory cells in the spinal cord being put out of action.
Without the controlling influence of these special cells
(which are called Renshaw cells) the motor cells produce
the uncontrolled spasms which may be fatal. Nowadays,
these spasms can be chemically blocked by using the drug
curare. While breathing is maintained by artificial respiration, life is saved by paralysing all the muscles for a few
days, after which time the inhibitory cells recover.

It seems likely that inhibition is involved in many aspects
of thinking. Take, for example, a well-informed person
being asked a difficult general-knowledge question. He may
often have to think very hard for ten or twenty seconds before
he finds the answer, which he then gives with confidence
that it is correct. What is happening during this period of
thinking? One possibility is that he tries one sequence of
thought and recalling after another, exploring one while
inhibiting others. In a slower and more conscious way the
chess player studying a position explores the various
sequences of possible moves, concentrating on one particular
line while other lines are inhibited. Inhibition is also involved in name-recall. Names from the past may be recalled
by following several different sequences of recollections.
Many sequences may have degenerated to some degree, and

no longer lead to the name, and a search must be made for another sequence that is intact and successful.

Clinical disorders sometimes exaggerate or caricature a normal mechanism like inhibition. There is a rare abnormality called cataplexy, in which the motor inhibitory mechanism is so much exaggerated that when the afflicted person feels a strong emotion even the motor processes involved in keeping him upright are inhibited. When he laughs heartily, the sufferer falls to the ground completely paralysed for a few moments, although quite conscious. The term 'helpless with laughter' is aggravated to an extreme in this condition. In such a case, the satisfaction of a good shot in a game like golf may have the same embarrassing effect. The disability can be very awkward, and often the victims adopt an excessively severe or forbidding manner in order to discourage people from telling them a funny story. No doubt the phenomenon of being 'paralysed with fright' is closely related.

Sleep-paralysis may also be caused by over-action of the inhibition mechanisms. In this disorder, an otherwise normal and healthy person is alarmed to find that he is completely paralysed on waking from deep sleep, and is unable to move for two or three minutes. This situation is frightening but is otherwise quite harmless. The process of sleep is quite essential for normal health, and it certainly involves inhibitory systems; it is probably significant that sufferers from cataplexy often also suffer from narcolepsy, in which the subject is liable to fall asleep several times a day, almost whenever he sits down in a chair. Doctors estimate that about 10 000 people in Britain suffer from cataplexy and narcolepsy.

Information processing in the brain

The method by which sensory impulses reach the brain is a very simple matter compared to what happens after those messages arrive. Let us consider the arrival at the visual cortex of a package of information from the eyes (see Fig. 10,

p. 53). This initiates a series of complicated events, a few of which seem to be as follows.

1. Most of the information is quickly discarded unless the brain is alerted to pay special attention. While the eyes are open millons of pieces of information must arrive in the brain every second, but unless the person is alerted to some part of this information, most of it seems to be rapidly inhibited and to disappear without trace. However, people vary in the extent to which they look around, and some have the habit of noticing a great amount of detail observed for no special purpose.

2. When attention is fully directed to one item, other items are often not noticed, and indeed their incoming messages may well be actively inhibited; but again, individuals vary greatly according to their interests, occupations, and training.

3. The image of the observed object is quickly processed for recognition. A familiar sight is often linked with a feeling response of, for example, safety or danger, pleasure or anger. The process of recognition involves a particular type of memory. We have many varieties of memory which often appear to be very different, but from the physiological point of view they probably all depend on similar mechanisms.

4. If the sight is unfamiliar and the brain fully alert, a life-long memory may be recorded that can be retrieved (remembered) as long as the brain remains in a healthy state. This storing mechanism is by no means an instantaneous affair, and the prolonged process of forming a memory will be discussed more fully in Chapter 8.

Information arrives in the visual cortex of the occipital lobes of the brain at a special receiving area, and the receiving cells seem to pass on the information very quickly to closely adjacent areas where various types of processing take place. Selected items are apparently passed on again to be correlated with, for example, related responses from the hearing areas (in the temporal lobe) and the body-sensory areas (in the parietal lobe). These intercorrelations seem to build up to what amounts to 'thinking'.

Thinking

The processes of thinking are difficult to define, and in no two people can they be exactly alike. In general terms thinking involves the linking and recalling of one memory with another and the forming of decisions for action. It may lead to conclusions or just to strong opinions—some stronger than others, and some worth more than others! Presumably the process of decision-taking is similar to the primitive decision-making process in relation to, say, running away from danger—similar, that is, but infinitely more complicated.

Man's complex varieties of thinking inevitably require the involvement of language, which is controlled by the dominant cerebral hemisphere. People suffering from speech defects caused by brain damage usually find that their thinking also is much confused—and to a much greater extent than in those suffering from injuries to the non-dominant cerebral hemisphere.

As old age arrives and new memories become ever more difficult to form, the process of thinking must inevitably become more dependent on old memories. Repetition may become more evident owing to the deteriorating recent memory. However, there is still the possibility that the older brain may contribute to existing knowledge by simply having the time to think, because the owner is less active than he used to be.

In general, man can think about only one thing at a time. It seems that when the brain is fully alerted—to something seen, heard, felt, or thought about—other matters are inhibited for the time being, and we are aware only of those that have links with the matter under consideration. These links (or associations) may emerge from any variety of memory store. Indeed, it seems that all parts of the brain may be involved in having even the simplest thought or making even the most straightforward decision.

The long sensory pathways

The better-understood activities of the central nervous

system are those concerned with the great pathways through which messages pass to the brain from all the special senses (Fig. 8), and the great down-flowing motor pathways from

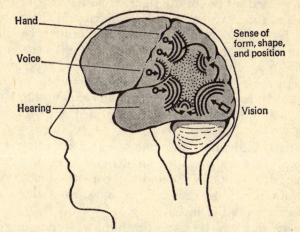

Fig. 8. The arrival of information to the temporal, parietal, and occipital lobes. This information seems first to be organized locally, compared with what arrives in the other cerebral hemisphere, then joined for more detailed correlations with the input from the other sensory areas.

brain to brain-stem and spinal cord, and hence to muscles. The parts of the brain from which these tracts leave and the areas where the great sensory pathways arrive are well known. The effects of small lesions (areas of injury) in the brain have been much studied and these studies provide extensive information about the areas concerned.

Damage to the cortex

Some of the early stages of visual processing can be disturbed by the effects of injuries near the visual cortex. It is interesting to study the resulting defects as they provide an insight into visual mechanism.

Destruction of even a minute area of the visual cortex of, say, the left cerebral hemisphere causes a permanent blind spot to the right of the point of eye-fixation in the visual field of both the right and the left eye, in exactly the same area of each. Destruction of all the visual cortex on the left causes loss of the right visual field for both eyes, although central vision is often unimpaired. This is called 'right homonymous hemianopia', and cannot be cured. Destruction of both the right and the left visual cortex causes almost complete blindness, which again is permanent, although the eyes themselves are normal and the pupils of the eyes still contract briskly on sudden exposure to light— this is a brain-stem reflex not connected with the visual cortex.

Similarly (although damage to one auditory cortex in the temporal lobe often causes no detectable disturbance of hearing) destruction of the auditory cortex on both sides of the brain results in complete deafness, even though the inner ears are quite intact.

Where the left cerebral hemisphere is dominant for language, an injury to this hemisphere may block the visual contribution to speech, and this results in the loss of all ability to read (termed 'alexia'). Print is seen clearly and vision is intact, but the words convey no meaning. However, other parts of the speech mechanism may be unaffected.

The failure to recognize something that is quite familiar is an important feature of some such localized areas of brain damage, and the effects may even result in a general failure to recognize familiar people, places, and objects. If there is some injury also to the right side of the visual cortex (in addition to injury to the left side) these disorders of recognition are often much more severe, and may lead to great confusion about the relative positions of objects, people, and places, confusion between right and left, or inability to find the way from one familiar room to another —a severe type of visual disorientation. At a more psychological level, visual imagery may be lost; the patient can no longer picture things 'in the mind's eye'. A man to whom this had happened, on returning from the Middle East in a hospital ship, told me he was looking forward to seeing what his wife looked like! The capacity for visual imagery is physiologically related to the visual content of dreaming, and after injury to the right side of the visual cortex dreaming during sleep may cease.

Similar disorders occur as a result of small injuries in other great receiving areas of the cortex. Thus lesions near the left auditory cortex may produce word-deafness, a condition in which spoken words are clearly heard but convey no meaning.

Damage to the sensory cortex in the hand area of one cerebral hemisphere affects the hand on the opposite side (see Fig. 9). After such injuries the subject can still feel

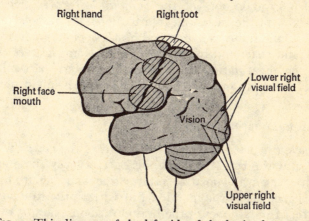

Fig. 9. This diagram of the left side of the brain shows areas of the cortex of the *left* cerebral hemisphere when injury leads to severe disorder of movement, control, and feeling of the *right* foot, the *right* hand, and the *right* side of the face and mouth, thus indicating areas of the brain controlling these parts of the body. The way in which one side of the brain controls the opposite limbs and opposite half of the body may have developed because all visual information is led into the brain reversed, as in a camera. This reversing is not only from right to left, but also from top to bottom.

pain, touch, heat, and cold with the affected hand but cannot recognize objects by touch, or localize the part touched, or even recognize the position of his fingers or arm without looking. Manual skills are also largely lost even though the fingers can still be moved, so that, for example, writing is impossible if it is the dominant hemisphere that is damaged.

As long as a hundred years ago, by studying such injuries neurologists were beginning to get glimpses of the localized functions of the brain. On drawings of the brain they attempted to identify centres for reading, writing, speaking, hearing words, etc. These diagram-makers in their own way made a substantial contribution to a difficult problem, but their diagrams have now been discarded as a naïve simplification of an extremely complex structure.

It is now known that the parietal, temporal, and, greatest of all, occipital lobes of the cerebral cortex receive the great mass of the incoming information: the parietal from the body and limbs; the temporal from the organs of hearing, smell, and taste; and the occipital lobes from the eyes. The language organization areas of the brain are particularly difficult to study and will be discussed further in Chapter 5.

The frontal lobes

We have discussed so far the behaviour of the cortex which surrounds the cerebral hemispheres, especially those areas which receive and analyse information arriving from the special senses and the muscles. But what is the function of the great frontal lobes of the brain? A vivid example of the controlling power exerted by our frontal lobes is given by the famous American crow-bar case of a century ago.

Phineas Gage, aged twenty-five, had a thick iron bar forced through his head by an accidental explosion. The bar entered like an arrow below his left eye and came out of the top of his head. He was stunned for only an hour, and then walked with help to see a surgeon. Quoting from a medical journal of the time: 'Gage lived for twelve years afterwards; but whereas before the injury he had been a most efficient and capable foreman in charge of labourers, afterwards he was unfit to be given such work. He became fitful and irreverent, indulged at times in the grossest profanity, and showed little respect for his fellow men. He was impatient of restraint or advice, at times obstinate, yet capricious and vacillating. A child in his intellectual capacity and manifestations, he had the animal passions of a strong man.'

The frontal lobes, like the cerebral hemispheres, are blanketed by the cortex, and have free communication with all parts of the brain, but especially with those parts concerned with primitive reward and drive systems, particularly in brain-stem, hypothalamus, and pituitary-gland regions (all situated at the back of the head, where it joins on to the neck). The frontal areas seem to provide a sophisticated development of these powerful survival mechanisms, and in so doing they seem to have acquired a controlling position over 'personality' and all kinds of personal decisions.

These functions are difficult to study, but they are demonstrated by the results of frontal-lobe injury. Slight injury may cause little disability, but severe injury has noticeable effects. It would seem that severe injury to the frontal lobes in infancy makes useful progress in education almost impossible, whereas in the mature adult the effects are different though no less dramatic. In the adult, well-formed habits of behaviour, stores of knowledge, and the ability to speak and read remain largely intact, and superficially the victim may appear to be fairly normal, but to his close friends he often seems to be quite a different person—his personality has changed, his mind has become unreliable, and certain dormant character traits may have become objectionable. This troublesome state of affairs is referred to as the frontal-lobe syndrome; it commonly appears after severe frontal-lobe disease or injury, especially if both sides of the brain are involved. Such an injury was received both by the unfortunate Phineas Gage and the soldier mentioned below.

A private soldier I knew received a severe right frontal wound in August 1944, but was reported to be conscious thirty hours later. He was rational a month after wounding, and there was no weakness of the limbs. However, after his discharge in November 1944, he failed to hold employment of any kind, and in July 1947 his father wrote: 'Since my son's discharge from the army he has shown no power of concentration whatsoever. He is unable to remain still for any length of time, walking from room to room. He sleeps abnormally long hours, and has an enormous appetite. He shows no interest in any hobby, and never completes anything he may start. His language is obscene, and his chief conversation is about sex; this began from his first conscious moments in hospital, when he said that all the nurses were prostitutes. Notwithstanding the fact that sex predominates in his mind, he has not shown any zeal or over-interest in running after girls, and I have no reason to think that I should have any worry from this. Books that he reads are of jungle subjects, and he only reads them at odd chapters, never from beginning to end.' The symptoms described here are typical of adult frontal-lobe injuries.

Surgical operations to destroy parts of the frontal lobes were introduced in the 1930s in an attempt to relieve a variety of personality disorders, after 'successful' operations had been carried out on neurotic chimpanzees. There is no doubt that such destructive procedures may greatly relieve abnormal mental distress, but the cure is at some cost in terms of loss of mental efficiency, and these operations are no longer regularly performed.

Hypnotism and pain

The response to hypnotism and the response to pain seem to be closely interconnected in the human brain, and it seems likely that the origins of both these responses lie in the region of the frontal lobes. There is no conclusive evidence that the pattern of reaction to pain is greatly altered in patients who have had major operations performed on their frontal lobes. The nature of the alteration, however, is rather surprising and will be discussed at greater length in the next chapter.

It has been reported that it is very difficult to hypnotize a person after major injury to, or an operation on, the frontal lobes. I have already put forward the suggestion that some people seem to have 'two minds', and if this is so then such people should be highly suggestible and easy to hypnotize. Thus it might be argued that the manipulation of two minds in such persons is only possible if both frontal lobes are more or less intact.

Yoga

It would seem that the now increasingly studied practice of yoga has some connection with hypnotism or, rather, self-hypnotism. A Yogi can control at will heart-beat, respiration, and his response to pain, probably by controlling hormone secretions. During meditation the Yogi hypnotizes himself into a state where all his metabolic processes operate at perhaps a quarter of the normal rate. Presumably those who effectively practise the meditative forms of yoga must also possess healthy, undamaged, frontal lobes.

4

Mind over matter

The commonly used phrase 'mind over matter' implies that mind is not matter. But the brain is now known to have such a complex structure that the 'mind' may well be matter just as much as is the rest of the body.

Pain

The sensory channels from all parts of the body to the brain incorporate an effective alarm system which warns of danger from injury, disease, or other emergency. This guard system sends very unpleasant messages to the brain which demand evasive action; these messages produce a response which we describe as 'pain', and the distressing emotions which go with it.

From each of the thirty-two segments of the spinal cord a motor and a sensory nerve root emerge which join together and then mingle with other roots to form the many nerves which supply and activate all the muscles and organs of the body. These nerve roots also provide a massive sensory channel from all parts of the body to the central nervous system. This vast system is much concerned with feeding back the information required to control muscular activity and bodily functions, and it also transmits the 'pain' impulses. The emotions connected with these impulses seem to originate partly from the frontal lobes. They seem to be different for each individual, so that there is no accurate way of comparing one person's feeling of pain with another's.

The amount of distress caused by pain seems to depend

greatly on the acquired characteristics of the individual. The brain has to decide for each experience, pleasant or unpleasant, whether it should be encouraged (repeated) or discouraged—to put it crudely 'it is the burnt child who fears the fire'. It is quite clear that parents who respond emotionally rather than practically to their children's minor injuries are in fact encouraging a reaction that will lead to their children suffering much more from the painful experiences of life.

A few children, especially in large families, learn to have a pain in order to get more attention. This tendency may persist for life, and some statistical studies have shown that the adults who haunt pain clinics tend to be members of large families. Every doctor has patients who for years complain of excruciating or unbearable pain, although they always appear to be in good health and never to have any relevant disease. However, it seems that the brain has the capacity not only to exaggerate suffering but also to do the exact opposite, by blocking all appreciation of pain through a process of 'auto-suggestion' or self-hypnotism.

On the other hand, in the assessment of medical and surgical emergencies, an exact description of the character, position, and effects of pain are often of vital diagnostic importance, while the intelligent layman's attempt to explain rather than describe his own troubles only complicate the issue. In my experience, Scottish miners are the best at giving a straightforward and accurate account of their symptoms, whereas Oxford dons are the worst. There are so many factors involved in chronic painful conditions that the therapist may do well to look on the problem as a game of chess between himself and the patient's health.

Operations to destroy a part of both the frontal lobes of the brain have successfully relieved persistent and distressing pain. After such an operation, it is said to be very difficult to hypnotize the patient, thus rather contradicting the connection between hypnosis and relief of pain (unless the operation has destroyed the systems that might have been relieved by hypnosis). The remarkable modification of painful experiences following these operations serves to illustrate the difficulty in defining what pain really is. It seems that sensory stimuli to the brain still arrive there and can be accurately described, but the patient to a large extent ignores the painful sensations and probably will not refer to them unless questioned specifically as to their severity.

Another strange pain phenomenon displayed by patients after operations on their frontal lobes is their violent reaction to sudden pain, though chronic discomfort does not trouble them at all. It is reported that women who have had the operation treat the first stage of labour in childbirth in a gay, cavalier manner, but over-react so vigorously to the second stage that special measures are needed for their control. In these patients the pain-feeling thresholds have been raised, but when the threshold is reached an uninhibited response develops. Thus the frontal lobes seem to have at least two somewhat conflicting effects in relation to pain. First, they can increase suffering by the emotional 'build-up' which they may engender and, secondly, they may have an inhibitory effect which damps down the uncontrolled response to an unpleasant stimulus.

It is well known that discomfort in one part of the body will reduce a feeling of pain originating in another part. It is widely believed that local heat-treatment relieves pain by increasing the circulation, but it may be that the heat really produces a competitive stimulus for pain mechanisms.

Pain at point A is not the only thing that can reduce a feeling of pain at point B; many other cerebral activities can also distract the attention. Listening to music, concentration on a game, or even puzzling over mental arithmetic will raise pain thresholds, and we are all familiar with the value of reading a story to a sick child, or grasping the arms of the dentist's chair in order to forget the pain of an extraction. Indeed, such procedures have been shown scientifically to reduce the pain experienced. The distractions of work and physical activity greatly raise these pain-distress thresholds, so much so that inactivity has an entirely harmful effect on many painful states. Indeed the tendency of modern civilization to encourage soft-living lowers pain thresholds and thus increases the sum of human suffering. If we abandon our comforts for an assault course in the army or for heavy labouring, our thresholds for pain and discomfort are at least temporarily raised in consequence.

Recently, a variety of stimulating actions have been shown actually to block the nerves in the spinal cord that are concerned with conducting pain impulses. These stimuli are most effective if applied to the skin near to the spot from which the pain seems to be coming. Electrical or vibratory applications may act in this way, and presumably acupuncture also, though the anatomical ideas behind this ancient method bear no relationship to modern anatomical knowledge, except inasmuch as the most effective places to insert the needles seem to be those where there is a high concentration of important nerves.

There are a number of relatively benign but painful conditions connected with muscles and joints that tend to build up a state in which a muscle in spasm causes great pain, which in turn prevents the relaxation of the muscle. This 'vicious circle' can be effectively broken by a variety of local treatments such as injecting local anaesthetic, applying a vibrator (electrical massager), manipulation, or the insertion of needles. Any one of these methods can often provide great and instantaneous relief, but resting in a position which relaxes the muscle in spasm often has the same good effect.

In some people severe pain can be self-induced by a certain type of apprehension, for example when the person concerned thinks of something unpleasant happening to someone else, such as a finger-nail being torn off or a small child falling heavily on a stone floor. (A similar effect is that of an expectant father experiencing 'labour pains'.) The pain often appears to come from the lower spine or the back of the thighs. It is by no means constant and probably occurs most frequently in people who have developed a sympathetic interest in others. People who do not experience a pain in these situations may feel their 'teeth on edge' or experience a cold feeling down their backs.

The fact that some people experience actual pain purely as a result of having a particular thought indicates the importance of emotion in relation to pain and suffering. Pain often causes a reaction of fear, and the apprehension which leads to a pain in the back or thighs is presumably a form of fear which can be deeply rooted in the past. Thus a woman who had been a 'problem' child experienced pain in her back when she feared that some of her misdemeanours were going to be found out. That the sense of fear in certain circumstances may lead to pain presumably strengthens the value of pain as a primitive signal requiring action for self-preservation. For if both pain and fear act on the same part of the brain no doubt they are capable of facilitating each other.

Phantom limbs

After a limb amputation many patients are frightened to find that they are conscious of the missing part. This is known as the 'phantom limb' effect; some patients even try to walk on the missing foot or grip with the missing hand. From a psychological point of view it is best if the surgeon discusses this problem with the patient in a matter-of-fact way, lest the victim develops any strange related delusions or symptoms. For example, Lord Nelson is said to have been conscious of his left hand after he lost his arm, and thought that this provided evidence that his body would one day be resurrected complete with the missing limb.

A particular area of the brain (the posterior parietal lobe) is trained throughout life to correlate the position of various parts of the body to each other and to their environment. This is referred to as the 'body-image' mechanism, and when one side of the parietal lobe is severely damaged by disease there is a lack of awareness of the other half of the body.

Provided the body-image mechanism remains intact after amputation, it still feels the various sensations coming up from the stump as though they came from the absent limb. If a child loses a limb at a very early age, before the body-image mechanism has developed, phantom-limb sensations are not reported. A phantom limb has been known to disappear after damage to the parietal lobe of the opposite cerebral hemisphere put the body-image mechanism out of action.

The phantom limb may be felt in its entirety, but more commonly the patient is conscious only of certain parts, chiefly those which during life were most highly trained in precision and sensibility. Thus after losing an arm the amputee generally feels the thumb and forefinger most often, followed by the remaining fingers, the palm, the wrist, the elbow, and the forearm. In the leg, the big toe is most often felt, then the remaining toes (which may not be clearly distinguished) and the sole of the foot, the middle of the foot, the ankle, the knee, and the shin.

Phantom sensations are usually described as a tingling which positively draws attention to a particular part of the phantom limb. The rest of the absent limb may seem to be missing from the phantom. The position of the fingers or toes (usually half-flexed) can be clearly described, and many patients say not only that the phantom can be moved about by moving the stump but that the phantom fingers or toes can be moved at will. In other instances the phantom hand assumes an uncomfortable position which causes an unpleasant feeling of cramped rigidity. The phantom arm is usually slightly flexed, but in the leg, the foot and toes feel as though they are in the normal position. The knee may seem either to be straight, or bent at a right-angle, even when the body is upright.

Many peculiar descriptions have been given by amputees of the position and performance of their phantom limbs. The phantom generally appears to move with the stump so that their relationship in space is maintained, and one patient whose arm was amputated in the middle of his upper arm used to amuse himself by rotating the stump at the shoulder, thus passing his phantom hand through his own chest.

As the months pass after amputation the phantom limb

usually seems to shorten or 'telescope', so that the hand or the foot keeps its size but moves nearer to the stump, until the phantom fingers or toes merge with the stump.

After amputation the cut nerves start to grow at the ends and gradually form bulbous swellings which consist of a tangle of small nerve fibres; these are called 'neuromata'. Phantom limb sensations often seem to originate in the neuromata, and pressure or tapping over a stump neuromata will result in pain which seems to come from the phantom limb. Many unpleasant phantom-limb sensations can be temporarily abolished by blocking the nerve to the stump with a local anaesthetic.

The phantom pains are likely to be felt in those parts of the phantom which are most important from the body-image point of view, such as the big toe, the heel, or the knee, for these areas have extensive representation in the brain. The patient may complain that an old corn on the absent foot is hurting again; and where wounds have caused great pain, and perhaps emotional distress, before amputation, the patient sometimes seems to re-experience the pain of the wound. These painful reactions can be treated effectively by 'percussion' or batting of the neuromata (a form of therapy I myself introduced in 1943, which has been successful in many cases of painful phantom limbs). Repeated percussion or vibration applied to the stump neuromata renders them insensitive and inactive, so that they are no longer able to discharge impulses to the central nervous system to cause pain and resulting misinterpretation by the opposite parietal lobe of the brain.

One man I knew had been conscious of a phantom foot ever since amputation and aware of a very unpleasant sensation that his big toe nail was being twisted. He also found that the stump twitched at night. The stump was healthy, but there were three very sensitive neuromata. Treatment was started seven years later, and the patient learnt to abolish both the phantom and its pain by hitting the neuromata with a wooden mallet via a six-inch rod, the other end of which he pressed against the tender neuromata. If he treated the stump in the evening he could depend on having a comfortable night. When he was first treated, percussion for ten minutes abolished the phantom for about half an hour, but after two weeks one shorter treatment abolished the phantom completely for four hours, and all discomfort was eventually avoided by one daily treatment of five minutes.

During percussion of one of the neuromata this patient gave a vivid account of the temporary aggravation of the phantom sensations. These included re-opening of the old wound of his foot, followed by a sensation of blood welling up between his toes. Percussion of other neuromata caused a temporary sensation of the nail being lifted off the phantom big toe. He generally felt he could move the phantom toes, but after treatment by percussion this subjective ability to move the phantom disappeared.

Thus not only is the association with the missing limb remembered by the body-image mechanism, but also the pain which was experienced in the limb before amputation. Further, this memory is forcibly recalled by stimulating the ends of the nerves in the amputation stump. These cases provide vivid evidence of the powerful effect of emotion on a simple type of physiological memory.

Disturbance of the body-image mechanism can also follow irritation of the parietal lobe, causing phantom sensations. Wounds of the parietal lobe may be followed by focal fits which lead to a phantom sensation of, say, the opposite arm being in a false position or of the limb seeming to disappear, but I shall discuss phantom-limb sensations caused by brain injuries rather than by amputations in Chapter 7.

Psychosomatic diseases of the brain: hysteria

The neurologist is trained to study and identify the various disorders caused by diseases of the nervous system, whether in the brain, spinal cord, peripheral nerves, or muscles. He can quickly identify the nerve or nerves that are not working if they are causing weakness in one of the limbs or other muscles in the body; and he can recognise the difficulties in, say, walking or using the hands that are due to diseases of the central nervous system, deciding precisely where the lesion is situated.

A neurologist must also learn to recognize when a disability is not due to physical disease but is produced by action of the patient's mind (or one of the patient's minds —in view of my hypothesis of the two-mind concept). This he refers to as a hysterical paralysis or spasm, or just as a 'functional' disorder which can usually be quickly cured by suggestion or persuasion. The neurologist must be familiar with a great variety of hysterical disorders including coma, convulsions, paralysis, spasms, severe pain, blindness or double vision, and deafness or loss of voice. These gross disorders usually mislead the family doctor, who may make matters worse by hinting at the possibility that some serious disease may be developing.

Hysterical paralysis

The hysterical paralysis of one limb is a remarkable example of a functional disorder; it is often accompanied by loss of feeling in the limb, so that no pain seems to be felt by the skin.

If the muscles are in spasm, and the examiner gradually but forcibly overcomes the rigidity, the patient usually cries a little, not because there is any pain but because he was emotionally committed to maintaining the muscular spasm and paralysis. This confirms the diagnosis, and a few well-chosen words will often produce an immediate cure, since these subjects are very suggestible (and, incidentally, easily hypnotized). Recurrence can usually be prevented by a few carefully planned remarks to a nurse, medical student, or other onlooker, saying that there is no serious problem and suggesting *en passant* (as a camouflaged threat) that, if there is any sign of return of the trouble, some complex and rather unpleasant tests might be required.

This hysterical reaction can also be caused by the effects of severe anxiety, which can greatly aggravate disability.

If after careful examination the clinician can say to a frightened patient that he is quite satisfied there is no serious disease developing, then it is common experience that a dramatic improvement or even disappearance of symptoms may follow. In most cases of hysteria, however, there is a *belle indifference* to the disability, and indeed there often seems to be an emotional longing to maintain the disability. Obviously reassurance is worse than useless in this situation, but determined persuasion is often dramatically effective. In the past, medical teachers frequently used the mass effects of a crowded audience in a lecture theatre to hasten the cure.

For example, a neurologist teaching in a crowded lecture theatre might say, '... Now, gentlemen, this poor young lady has complete paralysis with loss of all feeling in one arm and hand, and yet we can demonstrate no signs of interruption of the motor or sensory pathways in brain, spinal cord, or nerve. Further, there are certain features of the muscular rigidity which make it evident that this paralysis is not due to organic disease, but is of "functional" origin and, as I shall now show you, can be easily cured. Here I have a device for delivering an electric shock to the paralysed muscles, and when I do this they will jerk into great activity. Then this girl will at once recover the use of her hand, and the loss of sensation will disappear at the same time.'

This type of mass persuasion, though very effective and time-saving, does appear to neglect the underlying cause of the hysteria, and it is now recognized that such treatment must take place in conjunction with a thorough investigation of the cause. But I have followed up a large number of such cases treated in this way, and in general the long-term records of renewed health were entirely encouraging.

There are problems with this sort of treatment, however, for in medical work only a few doctors are trained to recognize an element of *malade imaginaire*, and many hesitate for fear of making a mistake. The difficulty is that any sign of hesitation is harmful, for in order to bring about a cure the examiner must be absolutely confident and positive in dealing with his patient. Even where there is some lingering doubt, it is sometimes best to treat the disability as being entirely functional, and then to observe what happens; mistakes are taken care of by making an excuse to see the patient again for some other reason. All doctors have experience of effecting 'miracle cures' but this must, of course, be confidential and have no publicity.

I well remember a soldier who reported sick while on leave, claiming difficulty in walking. An experienced surgeon who saw him was horrified to find obvious wasting of some muscles in the legs. Fearing the development of some variety of 'creeping paralysis', the surgeon advised admission to hospital for further study, and when I saw the soldier soon afterwards both legs were completely paralysed. However, on examination, the paralysis was obviously hysterical and the muscle wasting was due to an attack of poliomyelitis in early childhood. In retrospect the surgeon's obvious anxiety had made matters worse and led to an hysterical or fraudulent exaggeration of the disability. The sequel to this little episode was that on the following night the soldier absconded from the hospital by climbing over a wall, and rejoined his unit.

Most experienced neurologists will admit to having made mistakes in diagnosis when the very early signs of a disease such as multiple sclerosis are complicated by a gross hysterical exaggeration of the disability. In these circumstances the neurologist may be mistaken in deciding that the trouble is entirely hysterical—it is essential therefore that those cases seemingly cured just by persuasion should be carefully followed up.

The faith-healer has no such problems, for he has no need to make a diagnosis and can treat everyone in the same way. This is highly dangerous in the case of those illnesses for which a quick and accurate diagnosis is vitally important. Like the faith-healer, the busy G.P. is surrounded by a jungle of psychosomatic symptoms, but he must always be on the alert to identify new signs of symptoms which indicate serious organic disease. And the patient for his part should note carefully the dangers of 'crying wolf'.

Diagnosis is made more difficult in cases of hysterical blindness because some degree of reliance has to be put on the patient's description of his symptoms. Most people are frightened if they have any trouble with their eyes, and because he is worried a patient quite often develops some imaginary loss of sight in addition to whatever symptom has appeared. Thus the examining neurologist may find loss of vision in one eye, for which he can find no adequate cause. Even if there is some damage to the optic nerve, it is not possible for the examiner to tell by looking at the optic nerve how much the patient can see. Hysterical blindness of one eye is quite common and easy to deal with, but there are difficulties when a functional exaggeration appears in relation to some real background disease.

To help diagnose hysterical blindness in one eye, I have developed a simple device to check quickly for this trouble. The test takes only a few minutes and consists of asking the patient to read various test letters with one or both eyes open. Coloured lenses and letters are used, and the climax of the test arrives when the subject, with both eyes open, reads from the test card letters which are in fact invisible to the 'good' eye. The examiner then covers the 'bad' eye, and asks the patient to read the letters again—which of course he cannot do. The test thus proves that the sight of the 'bad' eye is in fact good, and suitable remarks to the patient lead to a disappearance of this hysterical blindness.

A person with an hysterical disability is often given away by his lack of knowledge of neuroanatomy. For example, in the case of hysterical paralysis of one side of the body the patient may, when asked to put out his tongue, put it out to the strong side rather than the weak side.

Hysteria and the two-mind concept

When we consider the functional disabilities described

above, we can again consider the idea that suggestible people may have two minds—let us call them mind A and mind B.

It will be remembered that children have this capacity to escape into a 'second' (fantasy) world, and that many adults similarly can escape using their 'mind B', whilst their 'mind A' does a monotonous job. Hysterical disorders may arise from a similar source, mind B taking control of, say, the weak leg without mind A paying much attention to what is happening. This may be thought of as 'subconscious malingering', since the conscious mind is not deliberately shirking, but this is not the whole story if mind A has ethical standards quite different from those of mind B. This concept should be seriously considered in its relation to hysterical illness.

Mental diseases

In the light of current knowledge of brain mechanisms I think that a more constructive approach could be helpful in preventing some forms of mental disease, and that educational programmes should take this into account. Thus the development of severe depression may be related to previous encouragement of unsuitable ambitions, while schizophrenia might result from allowing the development of two strongly opposing minds.

Elderly and lonely people may brood over past memories, especially if they are not busily engaged in active work with an emphasis on the future. In this situation their dreams can become frightening and shift towards hallucinations while they are awake, which may in extreme cases result in the vicious circle of paranoia with delusions.

Malingering

This account of hysteria is not complete without mention of true malingering or fraud, perhaps to get higher compensation after an industrial accident, to qualify for a blind person's pension, or for draft-dodging. The distinction between hysteria and malingering may be somewhat delicate for, whereas the hysteric can be cured by bullying, the malingerer is a more formidable opponent.

Once I had to tell a middle-aged man who had been drawing a blind person's pension for some years that we had decided he was a fraud. He stormed out of the room in righteous indignation, but as a double check we had arranged a variety of obstructions between him and the door, all of which he avoided without difficulty!

Malingering is also used as a device to get a free bed and food in hospital. For example, one elderly character worked out for himself how to simulate the signs and symptoms of a haemorrhage affecting one side of his brain, and by this means was successful in having himself admitted as an emergency to many hospitals all over England. This condition is investigated by a formidable X-ray test which shows the blood circulating through the brain (an arteriogram). One neurologist, who realized what was going on, asked him whether he realized how dangerous these repeated tests might be. The old man replied, 'Yes sir, I look on this as one of the hazards of the occupation!'

Some people even go so far as to injure themselves in order to appear ill or unfit for some duty—a reluctant draftee may shoot off his trigger finger. Sometimes the results of more subtle self-injury fool doctors into making the wrong diagnosis.

Dowsing and water divining

The concept of two minds arises again in the case of water-divining (or dowsing). The concept might help to explain the surprising fact that the skills of the dowser fail under test conditions. Thus he cannot tell which of a group of closed containers is full of water nor can he operate with his eyes closed or if he is blindfolded.

Dowsers nowadays specialize in some subject, for example, identifying the best places to dig on an archaeological site. The procedure is as follows:

1. The dowser visits the site and carefully studies all that is known about it.

2. Some hours later he studies a map of the site and holds his divining pendulum over the map for a preliminary identification of possible spots. This can only be done with full vision and understanding of the problem.

3. He then visits the site on another day, endeavours to make his mind a complete blank and forget all about stages 1 and 2, and then uses the dowsing rods to identify good areas.

In this sequence, the expert apparently feels he is tapping some hidden source of guidance, but it can be argued that he is simply making use of the information rationally collected in stages 1 and 2. If he really makes his mind a complete blank perhaps this is mind A, and the initiative has been transferred to mind B. If this suggestion has any substance, then one would expect dowsers to be easily hypnotized and to lose their skills if the frontal lobes of the brain were damaged.

Miracle cures and diagnosis

I have already mentioned the likelihood that cures of hysterical illnesses may be regarded as miracle cures. All such cures and diagnoses should be seriously analysed, of course, and it will usually be found that there is some logical explanation—maybe in terms of 'mind A' and 'mind B'. Often the most interesting feature in the investigation of surprising cures is the personality of the patient.

The publicity given by the news media to miracle cures and the like can be especially dangerous. By this means a very large number of people were recently induced to try a new form of diet which had never been tested but was supposed to cure certain diseases. The theories put forward for this particular regime were full of shocking misconceptions, a danger which is always present when 'miracles' are extolled by the lay Press rather than experts, and against which we all should guard.

I remember playing golf in the 1930s with a distinguished barrister who later became Lord Chief Justice, and much to my astonishment, during the game, he proceeded to proclaim the wonders of the 'black box' as a major scientific advance.* That a brilliant lawyer can be impressed by a device which no scientist could take seriously, shows just how isolated we can get in our own spheres of thinking.

* This black box was an instrument devised in the 1930s which, it was claimed, could diagnose disease.

5

Sight and language

The simplest way to learn about the processing of incoming sensory information is to study vision in relation to the double brain (which was first discussed on p. 29). The anatomical arrangements are very precise, and the site and extent of any lesion affecting the visual cortex are easily identified by the symptoms. Similarly, the language territory may be investigated by studying lesions which cause speech defects.

The visual cortex

The visual pathway from the retina of the eye to both occipital lobes of the brain is shown in Fig. 10.

The double brain divides the visual information by a precise vertical division, so that all the nerve fibres from the right half of the retina of both right and left eyes go to the right occipital lobe, and correspondingly the fibres from the left half of each retina go to the left side of the brain.

These right and left halves of the retina are not much involved in central vision (as used for, say, reading), for which one very sensitive spot (the macula) in the centre of the retina is used. When we look directly at an object, as for example in reading, the image is projected (reversed) on to the macula, where the concentration of visual cells (photoreceptors) is much greater than in any other part of the retina. It is for this reason that an object looked at directly rather than sideways is seen in much greater detail.

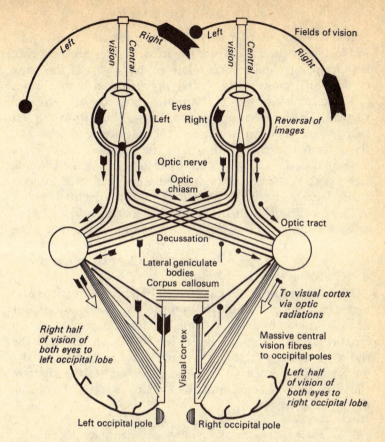

FIG. 10 Diagram to show the eyes, the optic nerves, optic tracts, optic radiations, and visual cortex (occipital lobes). Man's eyes face forward, and all objects seen are reversed by the convex lenses, as occurs in any camera. Owing to this arrangement, objects seen to the right of central vision activate pulses which pass to the *left* side of the brain for analysis. Both eyes see to both right and left of central vision, and from both eyes objects seen to one side activate pulses which travel to the opposite side of the brain. During the evolution of man, this arrangement of the visual pathways may have dictated the development of dominant control of movement and sensation in the limbs and body on one side by the opposite side of the brain. The reversal of images in the eye also takes place vertically, and this results in objects seen in the lowest part of the field of vision activating pulses which reach the upper part of the visual cortex. (The motor and sensory areas of the cortex are also 'upside down', so that the upper-most part of the motor area controls the opposite foot.)

Macular vision is necessary for reading and for all 'fine' work. The nerve fibres from the macular area are therefore very numerous and form a relatively large part of the optic nerve which conveys the visual signals towards the brain.

The macular fibres in the optic nerve are also divided vertically into two groups, so that nerve fibres from the left half of each macular area go to the left occipital lobe and those from the right half go to the right occipital lobe. The final pathway to each occipital lobe is called the 'optic radiation'. When the left optic radiation is injured, objects being looked at tend to be cut off from the right side, but in fact reading is still quite possible as the subject learns to look slightly to the right of the point of fixation. The macular fibres in each optic radiation go to the most posterior part of the visual cortex, at the extremity of the occipital lobe.

Macular vision is obviously very important, but it is also necessary that we should be able to see small objects out of the corners of our eyes, while looking straight ahead at a fixed spot. For example, if the left eye is covered and the right eye looks straight at a fixed spot, we can normally see a small object at an angle of about 90° to the right of the direction of gaze, and about 50° to the left of the direction of gaze.

Fig. 11. The region in the cerebral hemisphere at which the temporal, occipital, and parietal lobes all come near to each other is a specially important region for correlation and communication between the main receiving areas. Deep in this brain region, there also lies the optic radiation which is conveying information from one half of the eye. If the optic radiation is completely destroyed there results a complete loss of one half of the field of vision in both eyes. When this injury is to the left cerebral hemisphere, it is the right half of the field of vision that is lost.

When the optic radiation is only partly destroyed, the shape of the visual-field loss indicates which part is cut, and in these three visual field charts can be seen the effects of the destruction of (a) upper, (b) middle, and (c) lower parts of the optic radiation respectively. The thick black line indicates the extent of the visual field in degrees, and the restricted areas in the different parts of the right field indicate areas for which there is complete blindness—in much the same position for both eyes.

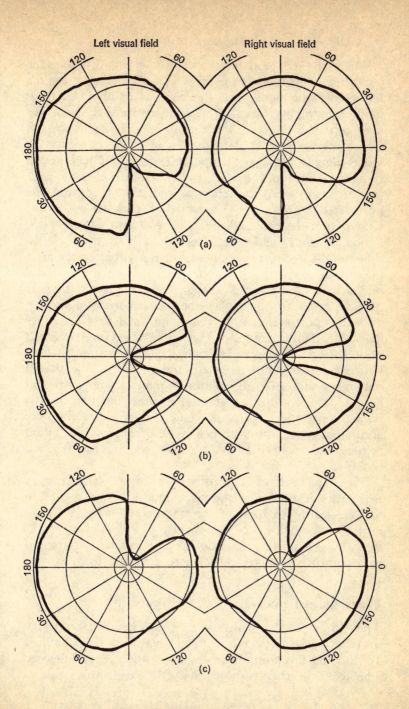

Left visual field   Right visual field

(a)

(b)

(c)

The right half-field for the right eye is called the temporal field, and the left the nasal field. For the left eye the left field is temporal, and the right is nasal. (The nasal fields are smaller—partly, but not entirely, because the nose gets in the way.) Thus the fibres arriving in the left visual cortex from the left halves of each retina convey visual signals from the temporal (right) half-field of the right eye, and from the nasal (right) half-field of the left eye (see Fig. 11). When the left optic radiation is injured, the field defect in the right visual field affects each eye in the same part of the field and to the same extent. This is called a 'homonymous' field defect (see Fig. 11).

Some of the changes occurring in the visual cortex after the arrival of visual impulses have already been mentioned (see p. 26). These complex changes take place extremely quickly, and the capacity of the visual cortex in dealing with an endless stream of visual information is most remarkable. Only a minute fraction of the visual input is noticed, and there must be some slight separation in time between looking at one object and the next. We should remember that, from the neurone's point of view, a period of one second is quite substantial in time—enough for 400 pulses to pass along its axon. Reliable details about rapidly occurring events are very poorly absorbed, so that visual evidence of events like road accidents is notoriously unreliable.

The exponents of impressionist art were quite correct when they insisted that the visual impression of a picture or scene conveyed little of the fine detail. Why bother to draw the detail if nobody sees it? In place of detail, therefore, the general impression of a scene can be exaggerated in a painting to increase the more dramatic features.

The language territory

The extent of the main part of the language territory (usually in the left cerebral hemisphere) has been defined by studying the positions of lesions causing speech defects. The area concerned is shown in Fig. 12; its centre is where

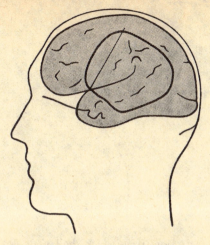

FIG. 12. The left cerebral hemisphere. The black line marks an area within which a small brain injury almost always causes severe disorder of the language function, temporary or more permanent, according to the exact position and depth. Usually such injuries also result in weakness with loss of feeling in the right hand and arm and/or a defect of perception in the right visual field

the parietal, occipital, and temporal lobes meet each other. It is here that the inputs from seeing, hearing, feeling, and moving are most closely connected to each other, and every facet of this arrangement has to be cultivated if the full contributions of speech to thought and of thought to speech are to be utilized. The different contributions to the language territory are shown diagrammatically in Fig. 13.

In most instances, an injury to any part of the language territory produces a profound disturbance of all aspects of the language function, along with considerable confusion. This general effect is often temporary, and no doubt reflects the close connections between all the areas of the organization in this part of the brain. Indeed, it is known that damage to a group of cortical neurones not only inactivates those directly injured but also temporarily inactivates neurones in other parts of the central nervous system with which they are in direct communication via nerve tracts.

Memory and learning depend on the integrity of a particular part of the brain (this is called the limbic system and will be discussed further in Chapter 8), much of which lies in the temporal lobe and well within the language territory. All aspects of language depend on the remembering of words, as also do the closely related mechanisms

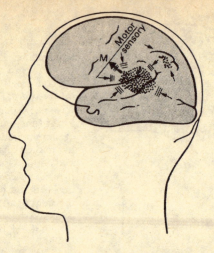

Fig. 13. The various directions from which the language organization is built up. The arrow going forwards towards the area M represents a stage in the production of the motor component of speech, and this requires the integrity of the lower part of the motor cortex at M. This part of the motor system controls the movements of the face, tongue, palate, and vocal cords and in the left cerebral hemisphere dominates the use of these structures for speaking. Small injuries to this part of the brain alone may cause a complete inability to speak, while the ability to read, write, or understand what is said is unaffected.

of intelligent thinking. Thus injuries to the limbic system or to its connection with the part of the cortex concerned with speech are likely to cause much more permanent disorders of language and thinking than do similar wounds to other parts of the language territory.

From the structural point of view, the left and the right cerebral hemispheres seem to be identical, but the special uses—such as language—for which one side develops in man provide opportunities to study cerebral mechanisms in special detail. If we now consider some more specific defects which can arise from lesions in the language territory, the examples should give a good indication of how all parts of the language territory act both interdependently and independently. I shall first discuss speech defects (termed 'aphasia'), and then difficulties with reading, wr-ting, and comprehension.

Difficulties with speech, reading, and writing

Motor aphasia

The production of appropriate words in relation to a considered situation requires that the lower part of the left motor area be intact (where the left hemisphere is dominant).

The victim whose brain is illustrated in Fig. 14 was a soldier who received a glancing blow from a bullet which penetrated his helmet. He remained fully conscious, but he became quite unable to speak and his right hand immediately became numb. However, his legs were unaffected and he walked two miles to meet the stretcher bearers. Fragments of bone were removed from the area of skull shown in Fig. 14(a) but, although he recovered sufficiently to return to work, his speech was still indistinct. After his death in a road accident some years later, his brain was examined and the small area of damage shown in Fig. 14(b) shows the scar of the previous brain wound involving the lower left cortex. The soldier's speech had recovered because, although damaged neurones can never grow again, other parts of the brain had taken over speech control, by a process of adjustment and re-learning. This cannot happen, of course, where there is extensive brain damage.

In some injuries that cause a mainly motor type of aphasia, the ability to read and write may be quite well preserved but the words spoken and written are nonsensical—'jargon' speech. Fig. 15 illustrates the writing of one such patient. There is a similarity too with impressionist art (mentioned earlier in this chapter), where by a few disjointed phrases the writer creates a vivid impression of the voyage described; although in this instance the effect is not contrived but is a direct consequence of the injury.

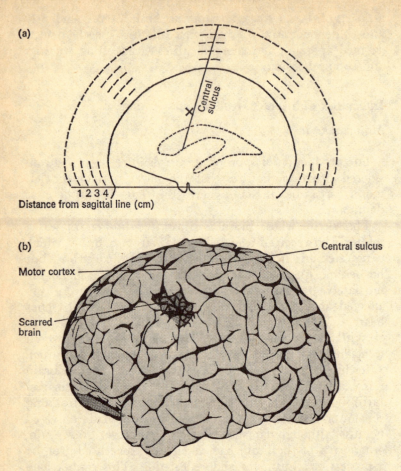

(a)

Central sulcus

1 2 3 4

Distance from sagittal line (cm)

(b)

Central sulcus

Motor cortex

Scarred brain

FIG. 14. (a) The position of a small wound which caused motor aphasia only. The site of the original wound was charted at X from the original radiographs of the skull. This small area is the lower part of the motor area which on the left side is specially organized for speaking. (b) Here the area of the old scar is clearly seen.

When aphasia is caused by a stroke, damage to the language territory may be severe and often paralysis of the right hand and leg, and loss of the right half of vision, may occur as well.

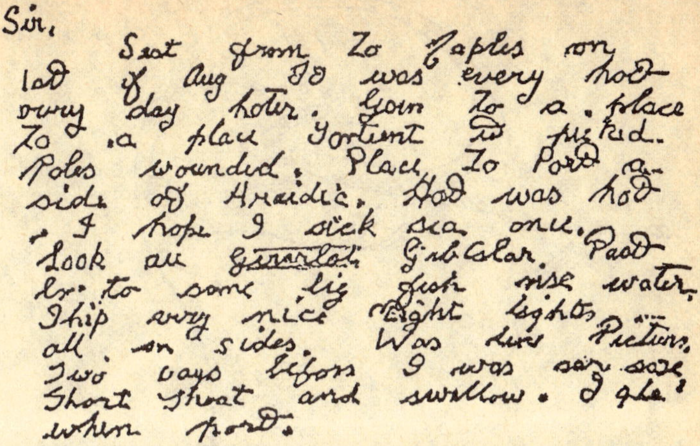

FIG. 15. Jargon writing produced by a patient two months
after sustaining a small brain injury.

Alexia

Loss of the ability to read is termed 'alexia'. It is often
associated with injuries involving the rear part of the left
optic radiation. The position of this is shown in Fig. 16(a),
and a typical injury causing alexia is shown in Fig. 16(b).

The special effects on reading caused by injuries of this
variety are not due to the damage to the optic radiation
but seem to be caused by direct injury to that part of the
brain which processes the visual input. It seems that this
processing can usually be done only in the left occipital
lobe of the brain (of right-handed people) and is an
essential prelude to the written information being of use.
This is important, for it seems to indicate that not only is
the left occipital lobe required for the original efforts of
learning to read but that, throughout life this area of the
brain remains a vital part of the mechanism of reading.

The soldier who sustained the injuries shown in Fig. 16
(b) was conscious a few hours after being wounded; he spoke
well but was slightly confused. The following day he was
alert and cheerful, remembering nothing of events during
the previous two weeks, which included twelve days before

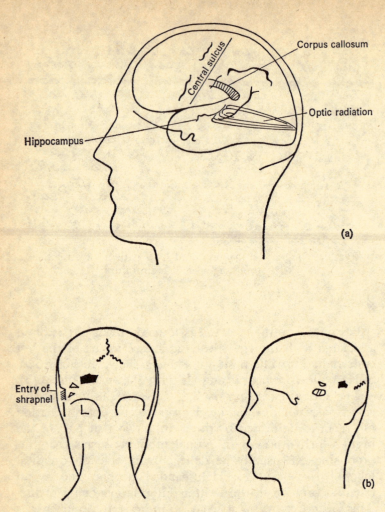

FIG. 16. (a) The position of the optic radiation in a lateral view of the skull. (b) The appearance of X-rays taken of a wounded soldier's skull immediately after injury and before an operation to remove the small bone fragments and the (black) fragment of shrapnel which severed the upper part of the optic radiation. The injury produced a defect in the lower part of the right field of vision, as well as a slowly improving alexia.

the wound. He carried out spoken instructions well, but reading was impossible and he could not even recognize separate letters. Reading continued to be slow and difficult, but he was able to work as a storeman after discharge from the Army.

In other instances where difficulty in reading is the most prominent effect of injuries to the language mechanisms, the subject may subsequently find impairment of visual memory and of his capacity for visual learning.

Mind blindness

Injuries to the brain above the level of the optic radiation produce some very unusual abnormalities, The patient can be conscious and able both to speak and read aloud correctly, but quite unable to understand what he reads. This rare condition is referred to as 'mind blindness'. Writing and spelling may also be a special problem resulting from injuries in this situation.

Agraphia

Writing difficulties are termed 'agraphia'. They are associated with injuries to the uppermost part of the parietal lobe, which is concerned with the preservation of motor skills.

Injuries to the upper parietal lobe may also bring about spatial difficulties, confusion between right and left, difficulty in finding the way in familiar surroundings, and loss of visual memories. As already mentioned, complete cessation of dreaming may also follow a parietal-lobe injury. This is to be expected if, as seems likely, dreaming involves the disconnected recalling of mainly visual memories.

It is vital for successive visual images to get out of one another's way, and a failure after injury of the mechanism which controls this function is very occasionally reported. The difficulties experienced by one victim included difficulty in finding his way and the loss of a rather special visual pattern that he had for numbers, days of the week, and

so on. Also there was a tendency for objects in his right
visual field to disappear if they were stationary, and
occasionally, during the early weeks after recovery, he continued to see an object he had been looking at after it
had passed out of sight.

Word-deafness

Inability to understand the spoken word (word-deafness)
is a feature of all severe cases of aphasia, especially if the
upper part of the left temporal lobe is severely affected, but
on very rare occasions word-deafness appears as a relatively
isolated abnormality. A disappearance of the knowledge of
foreign languages or a memory of music may also arise from
injuries similar to those causing word-deafness.

6

Concussion

Concussion is unfortunately rather a general term, as it is now used with more than one meaning. One common use is for a 'knock-out', after which there is full recovery and which is not thought to cause any real damage to the brain. However, the term 'acceleration concussion' is now used by doctors to describe the most common type of head injury. The effects can be slight or disastrous according to the acceleration to which the head is subjected. The human head, because of its bulk and exposed situation, is more vulnerable to the effects of acceleration concussion than is that of any other animal species.

The effects of concussion

Imagine a delicate clock lightly packed in a wooden box, and dropped from a height of five feet on to a concrete floor. This gives some picture of how dangerous it is for a man to fall in the street and strike his head. The velocity of the head on impact will be twenty or thirty feet per second; this movement will then be stopped, or even reversed, over a distance of a few millimetres. Thus for a short instant of time the skull is submitted to a very great and potentially destructive acceleration.

It does not need a student of dynamics to calculate which type of accident will cause most damage in acceleration concussion—consider what would happen if two motor cyclists were to collide head-on without wearing helmets.

The mechanisms through which the brain is injured

during concussion have been carefully studied, and it is now clear that the usual instantaneous loss of consciousness is *not* caused by cerebral compression, or by interference with the blood-supply, as was thought fifty years ago. It is now clearly established that the loss of consciousness is due to a direct effect on the nerve cells, and that this effect is related to the severe sliding and oscillating movements that develop within the brain at the time of concussion. These movements often develop at right-angles to the force of the blow, and the oscillations occur in opposite directions to each other in a manner that is known to stretch and tear nerve fibres.

These distorting oscillations particularly affect the white matter of the brain (see Fig. 5, p. 21), the deepest part of the cerebral hemispheres, which is packed with short and long tracts consisting of the axons of innumerable neurones stretching to other parts of the central nervous system. It is hardly surprising that these distortions to millions of neurones stop all brain activity and thus produce sudden loss of consciousness, so that the victim falls to the ground, limp and motionless.

Fibres in the brain or spinal cord which are torn by acceleration concussion cannot be repaired, though repair does take place when the damage occurs in a peripheral nerve. The severity of cerebral concussion is related to the amount of irretrievable tearing of the neurone fibre. At the worst end of the scale there is a permanent gross 'traumatic dementia'—the victim remaining helpless, paralysed, and mute for the rest of his life. At the post mortem in such cases the cortex may be comparatively undisturbed, but the underlying white matter will have been torn to pieces over large areas. Even after slight concussion torn fibres can be easily identified in the brain, when the death of the victim from other causes makes examination possible.

Fortunately the brain has great reserves of capacity and, in young people at least, recovery often seems to be complete. A student can again attend lectures with profit, and even if there has been some loss of old memories he cannot identify the defect. He may notice that new learning is slower, but this happens in any case and inevitably after the age of about sixteen. Children have the additional advantage of a relatively elastic skull, which reduces the accelerations. However, severe injuries to very young children may be quite disastrous as they may inactivate both the drive and the capacity needed to mature and to learn.

Repeated injuries have an additive effect. The disabilities and early ageing of 'punch-drunk' boxers are the most common visible effects of such unfortunate injuries. Death or severe damage may result from acceleration concussion without the skull ever being fractured.

Other head injuries

Until the early part of the present century special emphasis was often laid on the presence or absence of fractures of the skull, on areas of cerebral contusion (or haemorrhage) visible to the naked eye, and, of course, on the possible compression of the brain by haemorrhage from a torn artery. These are all important complications, but more basic, even though it is invisible to the naked eye, is the neuronal tearing that always results from acceleration concussion.

On the other hand, crushing head injuries can fracture the skull so severely as to tear cranial nerves without causing any loss of consciousness. The victim of such an accident often remains fully conscious, gets up, and walks away with blood pouring from his ears and nose because of the skull fractures. In one strange incident, the onlookers were so puzzled by this occurrence that they tried to wash out the bleeding ear with water from a bicycle pump!

A small object that strikes the head at a high velocity will cause a quite different type of injury. Injuries to the head caused by a golf ball are notoriously treacherous, for they may crack the skull over an artery without disturbing the victim's consciousness. Then, after a lucid interval, there may develop severe headache and drowsiness caused by compression of the brain by haemorrhage from a torn artery just below the skull. This situation requires operation within a very few hours if life is to be saved.

The shrapnel of modern warfare scatters small metal fragments at high velocity. If these strike the skull either they cut through the bone and penetrate the brain, or they bounce off, causing an explosive effect at the point of contact which drives a small shower of skull fragments into the brain. These wounds may cause no disturbance of consciousness, but the victim is often puzzled by the sudden effects in other parts of his body. A wound of this type in the parietal area on the right side might make him feel that his left arm has disappeared, and perhaps been shot away. Then when he sees that his arm is still there, he finds that it is, for the time being, completely paralysed and insensitive. Similarly a wound of this type at the back of the skull (the occipital region) will almost always cause temporary blindness with or without some permanent defect in the visual fields.

The treatment of skull and head injuries

All these penetrating brain wounds require early surgical treatment. In general, all the indriven fragments of bone must be removed, although often the metal fragment has either glanced away or penetrated deeply to lie in another part of the brain, where it can usually be left alone. Such remote fragments often cause no trouble as they were sterilized by their own high temperature at the time of the explosion. The surgical treatment of these injuries was brilliantly developed during the Second World War with the aid of the then-new antibiotics. The vast majority of the wounds were fully healed within two or three weeks of wounding, and where necessary a plastic or metal plate was inserted to fill a gap in the skull. Late complications such as brain abscesses and meningitis were very rare—in striking contrast to the high incidence of such dangerous complications seen after head wounds in the First World War.

In the 1920s and 1930s there was a firm tradition that

prolonged physical rest was a necessary part of treatment after head injury. During the Second World War, however, this was finally shown to be nonsense, and a vigorous programme of physical rehabilitation was found to be entirely beneficial.

Gradual recovery: amnesia

Although depressing, the study of head injuries has added considerably to our knowledge of the brain. Much can be learned from observing the stages of recovery from concussion, for in some respects the stages of development and maturation are re-enacted during recovery, which may take anything from a few minutes to many weeks, according to the severity of the injury.

Incidentally, the best basic guide to the severity of these injuries is the duration of unconsciousness, which may be a few minutes or hours, days, weeks, or years, according to circumstances, or of course the concussion may be immediately fatal.

Immediately after the blow, the whole of the central nervous system seems to be inactivated, and respiratory movements often cease. If recovery is to occur, breathing begins again and the reflexes return. Restless movements of the limbs occur and speech returns, at first with disconnected words or phrases. There follows a period of confusion, during which no two people react in the same way. Thus the victim may be drowsy or talkative, docile or aggressive, irritable or impudent. He may tell you his secrets, may be boastful or affectionate, and may even attempt to bribe his attendants to let him out of bed.

One almost invariable feature is that after recovery there is complete amnesia for this confused period. If, while confused, the patient is asked what the date is and what he was doing yesterday, he will probably describe events that could only have happened long ago, and will perhaps give the date as some years previously.

This period of confusion may last for minutes, days, or weeks, and then, often quite suddenly, the patient looks around and asks where he is. An interesting point emerges here; for it seems that the return to 'normality' depends very much on being able to put events into a continuous memory sequence as they occur. Thus for normal orientation it is necessary to remember what you have just said or done, whereas during the period of confusion the last vague memory may be of something that happened weeks or years previously.

The stages of recovery of consciousness, and particularly of the memory and speech functions, are of great interest. The following case record provides a typical illustration of the steps towards recovery from a severe head injury.

A shepherd, aged twenty-seven, was admitted to a hospital in which I was working on 3 May 1931, having been thrown off his motor cycle. When examined a few hours later there was no severe shock. He was bleeding from the right ear and was tossing restlessly in bed. He made no attempt to speak and was in a deeply stuporous condition. His recovery proceeded as follows.

4 May—Owing to violent restlessness he was transferred to the ward for incidental delirium, where he had to be strapped in bed. He powerfully resisted any interference and seemed very sensitive when his reflexes were being examined. There was little or no attempt to speak.

5 May—He fought hard against the straps which held him down and called out loudly without using any definite words.

9 May—He greeted me cheerfully with 'Good morning, sir,' and shook hands. He talked cheerfully about having to get home that night. Much of what he said was meaningless, but a few sentences were intelligible. He gave his name correctly, but in reply to a question said 'I've been here two years.' Sentences often began correctly, but later became meaningless: 'Here, could I go out into the ...' He almost wept when prevented from getting up, and seemed very annoyed. 'Well, I'll come back again,' he would say impatiently. 'That's no kind of way to ... now don't you think it.' Then, sitting up and waving his arms about, he would argue vehemently but quite meaninglessly with the attendant, and wept when again prevented from getting up.

19 May—He was very talkative and emphasized all he said with powerful gestures. He argued that he must go home, and boasted freely of his great skill at shearing sheep and catching trout. He promised to give money to his hospital attendants if they would let him go. He talked incessantly and repeated his arguments over and over again. Most of his sentences were coherent, but a few were meaningless. He paid little or no attention to what was said to him, and would not listen to reason. He had no knowledge of where he was and absolutely no comprehension of his condition. After considerable persuasion, he would respond to a simple request, such as 'Put out your tongue.'

25 May—He was quite changed. He remembered being troublesome in the ward and was now very apologetic. He said he felt very well and strong enough to start work again. He knew where he was and why he was there, and had a normal understanding of his environment. There was no repetition of his former unbalanced talk. He listened to and appreciated all that was said to him. He could not recollect certain events preceding the accident. He remembered driving along the road at a speed of about thirty-five m.p.h., anxious to get home before dark, and remembered actually colliding with the tar barrel which caused his accident.

Thereafter this patient's recovery was uneventful. When seen seven months later he was physically fit, but his doctor said he was much less reserved than before the accident. He had now no recollection of hitting the tar barrel, but remembered events clearly to within a few minutes of the accident. He was unable to remember the number of sheep he counted about six hours before the accident, but otherwise he could find no fault with his memory.

After becoming orientated to time and place, the victim can usually quickly arrange the events leading up to the accident, but there is almost always a period immediately preceding the concussion for which no memory can ever be recovered. This is called 'retrograde amnesia' and often involves only a second or two, if the victim was fully alert and awake when the injury occurred. Similarly, after recovery of full consciousness the patient usually finds he has no recollection of the period after the injury—the period of confusion—and this is called the 'post-traumatic amnesia'. For example, when a severely concussed motor-cyclist leaves hospital, he often has no unpleasant memories of the effects of his accident, in fact he may go out and buy another, bigger motor cycle. If, however, he had smashed his knee into another vehicle without being concussed, he would have memories of very great pain, so much so that he may well sell his motor cycle.

The retrograde amnesia is in most cases for a few moments only. The motorist remembers approaching the cross roads, the cyclist remembers losing control on a steep hill, or the window-cleaner remembers losing his balance. It is common in street accidents for the victim to remember being struck by a vehicle, but nothing more. His head injury may well have been due to his striking the ground a second or two later, so that in fact he is suffering a momentary retrograde amnesia. This momentary amnesia is observed after injuries of all degrees of severity and presumably has a clear and uniform physiological basis.

In some cases there is no retrograde amnesia. A quarryman was injured by a stone, about the size of a man's fist, which fell from a height of about sixty feet and fractured his skull. When questioned ten days after the injury he said that he remembered hearing the stone falling, and he ran to get out of the way. Then he remembered clearly a dull, crushing sensation in his ears, but nothing more until he came to himself in hospital twenty-four hours later. He did not remember falling to the ground after being struck, but the ground was soft, so that it is unlikely that he had a second injury while falling.

A goal-keeper remembered diving at the feet of the opposing centre-forward, and deflecting the ball. He remembered seeing a boot coming towards his face, then a blinding flash, but had no memory of the impact. He came to himself in hospital over an hour later.

The observations reported in this chapter are of particular importance, for it is only in man that we can get these glimpses of the interplay between related brain mechanisms. The brief and permanent retrograde amnesia is easy to explain, for the sudden concussion interrupts the repetitions which are required for a memory even to begin to form. Similarly it is not difficult to understand why events occuring during the period of post-concussional confusion are little remembered afterwards.

During the gradual recovery of consciousness, while there is still some confusion, the retrograde amnesia is often very long. Sometimes the patient seems to have forgotten several years; he gives the date and his age as they were several years before.

A Polish airman was questioned three weeks after he crashed in 1941. He was still confused and said it was 1936, and when asked about war with Germany replied, 'We are not ready yet.'

A greenkeeper on a golf course, aged twenty-two, was thrown from his motor cycle in August 1933. There was a bruise in the left frontal region and slight bleeding from the left ear, but no fracture was seen on X-ray examination. A week after the accident, he was able to converse sensibly, and the nursing staff considered that he had fully recovered consciousness. When questioned, however, he said that the date was in February 1922, and that he was a schoolboy. He had no recollection of five years spent in Australia, and two years in this country working on a golf course. Two weeks after the injury he remembered the five years spent in Australia, and remembered returning to this country, but the past two years were still a complete blank. Three weeks after the injury he returned to the village where he had been working for two years. Everything looked strange, and he had no recollection of ever having been there before. He lost his way on more than one occasion. Still feeling a stranger to the district, he returned to work; he was able to do his work satisfactorily, but had difficulty in remembering what he had actually done during the day. About ten weeks after the accident the events of the past two years were gradually recollected and finally he was able to remember everything up to within a few minutes of the injury.

A soldier was injured in an air raid in November 1940. When first examined he was in a deep coma, with limp arms and legs. Recovery of consciousness was very slow, and he did not begin to talk until a month later. By March 1941 his mental state was still greatly retarded. The retrograde amnesia was for about six months, and he had no recollection of three months in the Army. He now remembered coming to himself in hospital in January 1941, when he had found two women and a man sitting at his bed. These people had told him they were his wife, his mother and a close friend. He remembered arguing with them and saying he was not even married, and that he was certain he had never seen the man before. He was now correctly orientated, but was later still very uncertain of the main facts concerning himself. He did all intelligence tests badly, and had difficulty in reading, but he was very cheerful and friendly.

By April 1941 the retrograde amnesia had shrunk to a few minutes, and he remembered standing by the guns on the night he was injured and that a few shells had been fired, but he did not remember any bombs; the post-traumatic amnesia—the period he could not recall—was about two months. He remained popular with the patients, but childish and slow in his movements, with periods of irritability. He was invalided out of the Army in May 1941, and returned to light manual work in February 1942. He found his right leg and arm 'untrustworthy', and his relatives said he was forgetful and hesitated in his speech.

As the retrograde amnesia shrinks, memories come back not in order of importance but in order of time. Long-past memories are the first to return, and the temporary blocking of relatively recent memory may be so marked that several years of recent life may be entirely eliminated. For a limited time the patient may re-live his childhood, a state of affairs reminiscent of the symptoms of senility in elderly people.

During recovery, therefore, the retrograde amnesia often

shrinks at a varying rate to a point where memory of subsequent events ceases abruptly. By the time the retrograde amnesia has shrunk to a few minutes or less the patient has usually fully recovered consciousness, and indeed a brief retrograde amnesia is often an accurate indication of mental normality. I have considered further these important clues to brain mechanisms in Chapter 8.

Patients recovering from concussion occasionally find that events which occurred immediately before the injury are remembered indistinctly during the period of confusion, even though there will be complete amnesia for these events after consciousness has returned in full. This blurred memory may result in the patient making false accusations, as in the following case.

An electrical engineer, aged thirty-eight, was riding a motor cycle when a dog ran in front of him and he swerved suddenly and crashed. He was brought to hospital and found to have a fracture of the skull and gross bruising in the left frontal region. When re-examined five months after the accident he reported that he was quite fit and had been working regularly for three months. He said that he had no recollection of events for a period lasting from two days before the accident to two weeks after it. There was not the slightest recollection of the accident itself.

However, when this patient was examined two days after the accident, he was often heard to say, 'It was a dog.' Six days after the accident he was in a confused but very aggressive state and said 'I am supposed to have had a smash, but it wasn't my fault. A dog flew at me, and I flew at it. The farmer's son turned on me and smashed me with an instrument in his hand. He is getting arrested today. The police have found the instrument: everything is turning out as I said, marks on the instrument and everything.' The accident was witnessed by several people, and the only connection the farmer's son had with the accident was that he accompanied the patient to hospital in an ambulance.

In another such case, a doctor motored home a boy who had fallen off his bicycle, and the boy subsequently told his parents that the doctor had run him down. This was proved to be a completely false accusation, and the boy's confused recollections had been further complicated by his parents' questions. After recovery it emerged that there was retrograde amnesia for ten minutes before the accident.

However, if the victim can describe correctly events that immediately preceded the accident which caused the injury, then there is no reason to doubt the reliability of the description given of the accident itself, provided, of course, that he is not just repeating what he has been told after the injury. This may be of medico-legal importance, as in the Merritt trial (in the 1920s), in which an attempt was made with some success to discredit evidence given by Mrs Merritt of events that occurred just before she was shot in the head. The unfortunate lady gave evidence while conscious some days after the injury, although she died later.

Confused conversation during the periods of the post-traumatic amnesia may occasionally give important information as to the cause of an accident, and air-crew rescue teams are instructed immediately to ask the injured pilot, 'What happened?' This vital information (if obtained) can never be recovered after the return of full consciousness, and this phenomenon presumably corresponds to the ability of the patient with Korsakoff's syndrome (which is discussed on p. 101) to retain the capacity to repeat, say, a telephone number for a minute or two, even though he later forgets it.

'Visions'

Patients sometimes report seeing 'visions' relating to the injury after full recovery of consciousness.

A porter at a picture gallery was standing on a tramway island when a motor-van passed the island on the wrong side, hit the porter on the arm, and knocked him down. He recovered full consciousness in hospital twelve hours later. During the following two weeks he could remember nothing he had done for a period of about ten minutes before the accident occurred. About two weeks after the accident the retrograde amnesia lessened, and he could then remember standing on the tramway island just before the accident. Four months after the accident the period of retrograde amnesia was unaltered, and he had absolutely no recollection of the accident or of the twelve hours which followed. However, for about a week after his admission to hospital he had had on many occasions a sudden vision of the huge motor tyre bearing down on him while he threw up his arms unable to escape. These visions occurred only during the week following the accident.

A soldier was involved in a motor-car accident. He was sitting next to the driver when the steering rod broke. Five months later, he had made a good recovery apart from some headaches. He had complete retrograde amnesia for about twenty minutes, and post-traumatic amnesia for three or four days. Under drug-induced hypnosis he talked freely, but no shortening of the retrograde or post-traumatic amnesia could be obtained. He did, however, recover an 'island' in the retrograde amnesia, during which he was sitting in the car reading a letter while they were travelling at about thirty-five m.p.h. He also thought that he could remember looking up suddenly, but had no recollection of the driver struggling with the steering wheel, nor had he any memory of the rest of the car journey.

About two weeks after the accident he had his first vision, and he had six of these in all, of which four were during the two months following the injury. The visions consisted of the sudden appearance in his right visual field of a man, and especially the man's arms, struggling with the steering wheel of a car. This vision lasted for a few seconds. It occurred only while he was completely at rest both mentally and physically, generally while sitting in an easy chair. On the first two occasions of the vision he felt frightened, and his 'stomach turned over', but in the later attacks he recognized the vision and there was no associated emotional reaction to it. He was naturally a visualist and had visual dreams during sleep, but he never saw this vision during sleep and had no dreams about the accident.

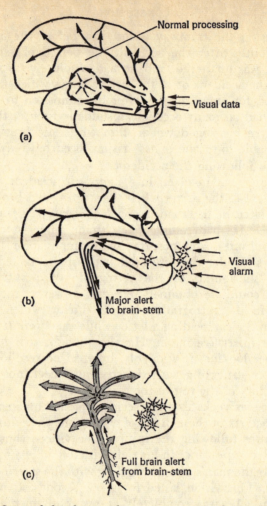

Normal processing

Visual data

(a)

Visual
alarm

Major alert
to brain-stem

(b)

Full brain alert
from brain-stem

(c)

Fig. 17. Some of the changes that seem to occur when, say, a motor accident causes severe concussion of the brain. These sequences are concerned chiefly with the visual system and are of great significance in studying memory.

(a) Visual information is being fed in normally via the eyes (from the right in the diagram) to the occipital region of the brain. Visual events are being processed in sequence and being correlated with previous visual experiences and memories.

(b) Suddenly some visual information arrives which, because of its pattern, appears to bypass the slower mechanisms, and sends an altering signal to the brain-stem.

(c) The brain-stem alerting systems respond with strong activation of all parts of the brain—a call to 'action stations'.

After this the following sequence takes place (not illustrated). (d) The accident occurs and causes severe concussion, during which all brain mechanisms are put out of action. Then breathing starts again and a gradual recovery begins—the pattern of this depends mainly on the severity of the brain damage and distortions at the time of the accident.

(e) If the victim is able to speak within a few hours of the concussion, he may be able to describe some of the events that occurred during (b) and (c), although he is still confused. These faint and temporary memories will then gradually disappear and become lost for ever. During this period of confusion it is impossible for these thoughts to be processed and consolidated as was occurring normally during phase (a) before the injury.

(f) The period of confusion lasts for, say, three days, and during this period no events can be processed for remembering and future use. This period is subsequently referred to as the period of post-traumatic amnesia.

(g) As full consciousness returns, the victim again becomes aware of the sequence of current events, and from now on can remember what is or has been happening since his recovery. These events may at first be difficult to correlate with the happenings before the injury and perhaps because of this there may be a period of months before the injury for which he has no clear memory.

(h) Naturally he now tries to remember what happened, and he succeeds slowly in remembering events before the injury—up to within perhaps thirty minutes of its occurrence. This interval before the concussion for which he can never recover any memory is called the period of retrograde amnesia.

(i) Although the period of retrograde amnesia remains impenetrable, during the first two weeks after recovering consciousness, the victim might occasionally, while sitting quietly and thinking of nothing, have a simple hallucination which is obviously a half memory of some very dramatic scene that occurred during phase (c) just before the concussion. These passing visions are not always associated with any emotional reactions. They become less frequent over a period of about two weeks, and then cease, never to return.

Fig. 17 illustrates the time-relationships between concussion, the stages of recovery, and the occurrence of various fragments of memory or visions about the accident.

During recovery from concussion there is also a striking connection between persisting confusion and long retrograde amnesia on the one hand, and the disappearance of all confusion and a short retrograde amnesia on the other. These significant relationships are considered further on p. 102 in connection with transient amnesic episodes.

7

Fits

Epilepsy has been a recognized condition in man for many centuries—it is well known that Julius Caesar may have been a sufferer from this disability. Epilepsy often begins for no known reason, but it also arises as the result of certain brain injuries or diseases, and a fit can even be induced in any healthy person by a suitable electric shock applied to the brain. It is surprising that we know so little about the factors that lead to epilepsy, and that even modern brain-wave studies have contributed so little to the understanding of the physiological problems concerned.

I think it is likely that epilepsy results from some imbalance between activating and inhibiting processes in the brain. This imbalance may have been caused by a brain injury received during birth or a serious illness: but sometimes develops in an otherwise normal brain and may be related to the complex processes of maturation and learning in early childhood. Epilepsy is usually treated by the regular administration of some anticonvulsive drug, which may be continued for years if it appears to prevent the fits from occurring. Many such cases begin to have minor epileptic fits in childhood, major fits often starting by the early teens. Epileptic fits that begin in adult life have to be studied critically, as they may give the first indication of some organic disease developing in the brain.

Major epileptic fits

A major epileptic fit (*grand mal*) is very frightening to

observe for the first time. There is often no warning of a fit before the victim loses consciousness. All the muscles of the body, limbs, and face contract violently to produce a rigid distortion, and the victim falls heavily to the ground, perhaps striking his head as he does so. Because the chest and throat are rigid, breathing is impossible, and the skin becomes blue from a lack of oxygen in the blood.

After perhaps twenty or thirty seconds of this violent spasm, short periods of relaxation occur, so that the muscle spasm becomes jerky (clonic). Because of the sudden contraction of the jaw muscles the tongue may be severely injured, by biting, unless some object is forced between the teeth to prevent this. The clonic stage gradually becomes less violent, then ceases, and breathing begins again; consciousness then gradually returns.

The physiological mechanisms involved are not well understood. All parts of the brain are apparently involved in such a fit, and the very sudden onset suggests the early involvement of a brain-stem mechanism. The similar spinal-cord convulsions of tetanus or strychnine poisoning are known to depend on inactivation of the inhibitory motor cell mechanism, and it is tempting to think that a major epileptic fit may have an analogous mechanism.

In most cases of epilepsy, however, the fits are separated by long intervals of months or years, as though a failure of the balance between action and inhibition slowly develops to a level that becomes explosive; in fact, there is often evidence of some type of 'build-up' in the days or hours preceding an epileptic fit. The fact that brain injury is one of the most common causes of epilepsy is perfectly compatible with this concept of a disturbed balance between two opposing physiological forces.

As will be discussed later, the fits that follow localized injuries to the cerebral cortex often begin with a 'warning', and may or may not progress to the *grand mal* just described. However, fits following local damage to the frontal lobes of the brain (see p. 32) tend to be of the *grand mal* variety with no preceding warning.

Fits induced by electro-convulsion therapy

A major epileptic fit may be precipitated in any person by an electric shock to the brain, and this is used as a form of therapy in some mental disorders. The effect of this shock is not instantaneous—as when a shock to a nerve stimulates a muscle to twitch—for the fit follows the shock after an interval of several seconds. It appears therefore that the therapeutic shock might break down a balance between the two opposing forces of action and inhibition in the brain in a manner that is quite decisive, for a fit always follows.

Minor epileptic fits

In the case of *grand mal*, the dramatic spasm, fall, and loss of consciousness dominate the picture, but minor epilepsy, *petit mal*, is a very different matter. Often the fit lasts for only a few seconds, and may be unnoticed by others. Usually, however, the subject stops whatever he is doing and stands still, with a vacant expression and perhaps slight muscle spasm of hand, face, or eye movements, then after a very few seconds recovers as though nothing had happened. He may himself be unaware of the transient loss of consciousness. Although this mechanism is very different from *grand mal*, here again, for a short time, most aspects of brain function are inactivated. It seems clear, however, that a different cerebral mechanism is involved in *petit mal*; the most likely mechanism seems to be some aspect of the part of the brain called the limbic system (which I will discuss in more detail in the next chapter).

The influence of the environment on fits

One interesting aspect of epileptic activity which has not been adequately studied is the probable effect of environment on the incidence of fits in those liable to convulsions (whom we usually call epileptics). There are many reports of children suffering from *petit mal* whose condition improves with a change of environment.

There is some evidence that, in some epileptics, a fit is unlikely to occur during periods of vigorous activity or mental concentration. It seems likely that certain types of brain activity should tend to counter the build-up to a fit, whatever the mechanism of that phenomenon may be. Thus there may be some other approach to the treatment of epilepsy which would be more effective than the current use of anticonvulsive drugs; but this has not yet been discovered.

Focal fits

As we have just seen, both *grand mal* and *petit mal* seem very suddenly to upset the brain *as a whole*, and for this reason some strange activation or inhibition of brain-stem centres seems to be involved at the start of the fit.

'Focal' fits are entirely different. They are suffered by people in whom a *small* area of the cerebral cortex is injured. The localized disturbances caused by the resultant fits are 'focused' in one area of the body and reflect the exact area of the cortex damaged. Therefore a study of these effects has enabled us to learn more about previously little-understood brain mechanisms.

Even though these focal fits may progress to a major convulsion, the localized warnings appear for perhaps half a minute before the loss of consciousness and can often be described, either during the first half minute or, more commonly, after recovery from the period of loss of consciousness. For example, injuries to the back of the head (occipital lobe) often cause a visual variety of focal fit. The most commonly observed of these takes the form of flashing lights in a blind part of the patient's visual field or a spreading loss of vision in a visual field that is ordinarily only slightly impaired.

The occipital lobes of the brain seem to be concerned almost exclusively with processing the vast visual input to the brain via the eyes, so it is not surprising that fits originating from lesions in this area usually have some visual symptoms. The remarkable variety of forms the phenomenon can take is presumably indicative of the complexity of the various mechanisms involved.

Each varying report of a focal visual fit gives a glimpse into a particular stage of the processing of incoming information, showing that this must involve aspects of speech, spatial sense, orientation, colour sense, and visual memory. Here are some subjective descriptions by one-time patients of mine, of visual warnings of a fit of this type.

—Flickering bright colours appearing in the left side of my vision, especially in the area where there is a defect in my vision.
—Live wires dancing in front of my eyes for a few minutes.
—Thousands of sparks of light whirling about in both my blind areas.
—Suddenly the blind half of my vision was filled with hundreds of tiny sparks of coloured light-red, blue, and green, moving downwards like snowflakes.

There may also be 'negative' effects.
—Suddenly everything looked as though it were far away and out of focus.

One patient lost vision in the left visual field, the loss lasting for half an hour. He then recovered, but during the 'spell' there was difficulty in recognizing objects being looked at. 'Everything looked distorted,' he said.

As we have seen in Chapter 5, total destruction of the optic radiation on one side causes a complete and permanent blindness in the visual field on the side opposite the wound. The optic radiation may be destroyed well in front of the visual cortex, so that this cortex is little damaged, if at all, but has nothing to do because none of the accustomed information can arrive. It is perhaps not surprising that an isolated piece of highly trained cortex might at times originate focal fits by way of 'rebelling' against this situation.

Damage to a small area of the right occipital lobe in one patient caused not only a complete blindness in the left field but also a tendency to focal fits with visual symptoms. The fits would begin with what he described as a yellow flashing light in the blind part of the visual field, which was followed in a few seconds by loss of consciousness and a generalized convulsion. In an attempt to stop these fits, the brain scar was exposed by an operation, and an electrically unstable area of cortex was removed—this was near the back of the temporal lobe. After the operation, the fits were less frequent and their character changed, for the visual symptoms no longer occurred. However, there was usually a *grand mal* convulsion without warning, so that in many ways the patient was worse off than before the operation. This case was particularly interesting because the visual warning in the blind field was eliminated by the removal of a piece of cortex situated well in front of the visual cortex.

One patient's brain injury caused permanent loss of the lower part of the visual field; he recovered well otherwise, except for occasional fits. These had no visual warning, but on the other hand, the patient reported a *continual* flickering of lights and colours in the blind part of his visual field, which continued unchanged even nine years after he had sustained his injury. In my experience this rare phenomenon does not usually become part of a visual warning to a fit, but seems to be caused by spontaneous activity of the occipital cortex. Normally inhibitory control would prevent it from reaching consciousness (see Fig. 18).

The most common of all the focal varieties of fits are caused by damage to the sensori-motor cortex. The motor warnings of these fits usually appear as jerkings (clonic movements) of one localized group of muscles in the limbs, face, or part of the opposite side of the body, without in the early stages disturbing consciousness in any way.

Focal sensory fits usually also develop in one small area, but as with other localized warnings, they often spread to involve larger parts of the body and then to cause a general convulsion with loss of consciousness. Among the varying sensations reported by sufferers are 'pins and needles', pain, hot and cold feelings, and feelings of being unaware of the position of one's limbs.

A great variety of sensations and movements may be felt during a fit. The symptoms of spontaneously occurring fits cannot as yet be interpreted with any confidence, but their

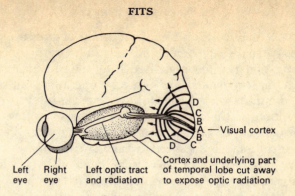

FIG. 18. Diagram of the visual pathway from left eye to left visual cortex (receiving area) at A. The brain areas designated B, C, D, etc. perform various stages in visual processes and in correlating with other parts of the brain. For example, if an injury divided the optic radiation and left A intact, the cells in area A might react by firing off a focal fit, producing an effect of flashing lights in the blind (right) visual field. This effect, however, can be recognized only if areas B, C, D, etc. are intact and can process and pass on to the brain as a whole the signals which are reported as flashing lights by the subject.

variety has given us some insight into the complexity of the functionings of the brain.

Of special significance is the occurrence of negative as opposed to positive phenomena in some focal fits. Thus if the hand is affected, it may jerk into spasm, or it may drop helpless: it may seem to move into a false position, or it may just seem to disappear as regards any sensation coming from it. Visual effects may involve flashing lights or just a spreading blackness. Or again in relation to minor fits, the sudden black of these episodes may well be related in an opposite sense to the vivid hallucinations that often arise from fits originating in memory systems (perhaps the limbic system) of the temporal lobe area. Further, in major epilepsy, the transition from a violent tonic spasm to clonic jerks and then to flaccid paralysis must be highly significant from a physiological point of view.

When epileptic fits develop for the first time in adult life, it is usually necessary to investigate the possibility that the cause may be a disease of the brain or pressure on the brain—perhaps by some kind of lump or tumour. This investigation is often organized in a department of neurological surgery where any necessary operation can also be carried out. As with the fits following brain injury, an exact description of the attack may indicate which part of the brain is being disturbed, and this is often confirmed by a demonstration of localized weakness, loss of sensation, aphasia, or change in the visual field, all of which are investigated in the routine neurological examination.

In addition there are several sophisticated radiological methods which can show the circulation of the blood through the brain and the position of the ventricles in the middle of each cerebral hemisphere. The investigations are thus made extremely precise. Often these tests can be completed at a leisurely rate, but when the pressure within the skull is raised, it may be necessary to act with considerable speed.

The actual operating procedure for exposing a large area of the brain has been greatly improved in the past thirty years, and is now remarkably safe. Often the chosen plan is to remove a slab of skull on one side, measuring perhaps ten centimetres square. A somewhat larger flap of scalp is first turned down from above in order to maintain the main blood-supply from below, and after the operation both the skull and scalp can be returned to heal in the normal position and thus to leave little or no visible scar after the hair has grown again.

Hallucinations and dreams

Hallucinations may be auditory (for example, the hearing of threatening voices), or visual, or even involving the senses of smell and touch. They may be caused by mental illness, brain damage, severe illness, starvation, or thirst, and are often linked with some previous thought or experience. Drug-induced hallucinations are found stimulating by some but unbearable by others. A drug user can usually describe in great detail hallucinations induced by, for example,

LSD, but the physiological causes of hallucinations are probably best investigated by studying the effects of brain damage.

The preliminaries to a fit may include hallucinations, whose nature is related to the area of the brain damaged. Fits which are due to temporal-lobe injuries may cause hallucinations involving vision, taste, smell, or hearing, whereas the hallucinations at the beginning of a fit caused by injuries in the posterior parietal and occipital areas seem to be mainly visual, but may spread to involve the body-image mechanism of the arm or leg, which is also known to be dependent on this part of the brain.

Visual hallucinations and hallucinations of self

When we look at an object, we must assess its position in relation to other objects around it, and to our own bodies. The position-sense of the body and limbs is a function of the parietal lobes of the brain and is learnt early in life. Near the midline of the parietal lobes there is a 'centre' controlling the specific reactions which cause powerful movements of the head and eyes to the opposite side. In its primitive form, if there is visual alarm in the right visual field, this centre causes a quick turn of the head and eyes to the right with a protective movement of the right arm. A protective movement of this kind is called an 'adversive' reaction.

Fits which develop after injury to both the parietal and occipital lobes, near the midline, indicate the close relationship of the vision, body-image, and adversive functions, as is shown by the following examples.

One patient had four types of attack: *grand mal* attacks without warning; adversive attacks involving the eyes and the right hand, which led to momentary loss of consciousness; a sudden shadow moving across the right half of the visual field, 'like a cat running across', without loss of consciousness; and episodes in which his right hand would suddenly seem to be raised up above his head—he would look towards it and seem to see it momentarily, and on occasion had asked his wife to pull it down. This fourth type of attack lasted for less than thirty seconds, and ended abruptly; there was some confusion during them, but if his attention was directed towards his hand in its real position the patient would admit to seeing it there.

Another patient's epilepsy took the form of sudden attacks in which his left hand looked queer and out of place; it did not appear to be in the place where he felt it. He felt the limb did not belong to him, and would waggle his fingers and watch them moving to assure himself that what he was looking at was his own limb. This sensation lasted for a few seconds only, after which he lost consciousness and had a generalized *grand mal* convulsion. On other occasions he had the preliminary symptoms only, without any *grand mal* attack.

Another example is a patient whose attacks were of two sorts. In one there was a sudden intense feeling of rotation, always to the right. If walking, he would be forced to veer to the right in a circle. This would last for a few seconds only and end abruptly. In the second and less frequent sort of attack he would have a sudden feeling of being detached from his body, so that he was observing it as if looking at someone else. There was a definite visual quality about the attacks—'I see myself as separate and watch myself from outside and slightly above me.' On one occasion this had led on to loss of consciousness and falling.

One very interesting case was of a patient who had a variety of epileptic phenomena. Soon after receiving a head wound he developed sudden *grand mal* attacks without warning. Later, attacks occurred in which objects he was looking at would suddenly fade out and be replaced by a black or grey spot, spreading to completely block the left visual field. This would sometimes lead on to a *grand mal* attack. In other attacks the left visual field seemed suddenly to be filled with coloured balls of light, and as he looked at them they changed to multiple figures of men. On later occasions he saw these figures and recognized them as multiple images of himself—tiny replicas which seemed to move towards him and then recede again; they were of the top half of the body only, and if he moved his arms the figures seemed to move theirs in a similar way. For a limited period of several days together he also had attacks of a sudden black spot obscuring his vision but, instead of remaining a negative phenomenon, the area was suddenly occupied by a life-size picture of a man's head and shoulders; as he looked, 'it suddenly dawned on me it was myself'. It was a mirror image, and again could be made to imitate movements he himself made. On occasion all of these hallucinations had been the preliminary to *grand mal* attacks.

In the last two patients' cases the mechanism for central integration of the body-image itself seems to be involved, but in two different ways. In the first, there was a visual impression of his own body-image from without, as if the visual and postural and movement elements of the vision had become separated. In the second, we see a gradual build-up of a hallucination generated completely by the brain, from what at first seems to have been a simple almost unformed focal visual fit.

It may seem surprising that a local injury to the occipital and parietal areas should be followed by fits which feature hallucinations of self. (It is interesting that these are from the waist up as often seen, and no doubt studied, in a mirror.) This type of fit must surely reflect some special feature of the subject's psychology. But there is also convincing evidence that the area of the brain involved is very much concerned with the storing of visual memories—for example, injuries in this area sometimes lead to a cessation of dreaming, and dreaming seems to be associated with a false activation of visual recalling systems, as in other types of hallucination.

Hallucinations of remembered scenes

Another result of damage in this area of the brain is vivid, formed hallucinations of remembered scenes. Often these visions are seen in that half of the visual field which had been defective or is still faulty.

One patient, in addition to attacks of intermittent red flashing lights in the right half of his visual field, would suddenly see in this field pictures of his experiences immediately after receiving the injury in which his brain damage was caused. He would see stretcher-bearers walking past, and then the figures of nurses whom he would recognize. The figures were smaller than normal and seemed flat and uncoloured rather like a black-and-white film. They appeared in addition to real objects seen in the left visual field.

In another case the visions were superimposed on the preserved part of the field, which was still seen clearly, producing a most bizarre experience. While in the cinema, this man saw in his right visual field various objects in his hospital ward. These appeared as a continuation to the right of the screen, to the left of which he could still see the film he was watching. The images were similar in colouring to the pictures on the film. On another occasion, while in bed in the ward, he suddenly saw a motor cycle and then a convoy of lorries passing from right to left in his right visual field. They appeared to be passing over the end of the bed, which he could still clearly see in his left visual field. On this occasion, the attacks proceeded to a *grand mal* convulsion.

Another man, in addition to attacks of clonic facial movement leading to adversive reactions of the left side and loss of consciousness, also had attacks in which he felt hot, his thoughts seemed to get out of control, and he felt as if in a dream that he was back in Khartoum during the Second World War. However, he could still see and recognize friends around him. This experience was accompanied by strong apprehension and frustration which exactly reproduced the emotions he had in fact felt in 1940 in Khartoum when he thought that he ought to be in England taking a more active part in the war.

In these cases it appears that the memory store is being activated directly by the epileptic process. The hallucinations which occupy only half the field of vision are, of course, associated with some damage to the opposite occipital lobe.

Hallucinations of smell, taste, and hearing

Epileptic fits arising from injury to the temporal lobes of the brain are often associated not only with visual hallucinations but also with hallucinations of smell, taste, or hearing. The hallucinations may also feature an intense feeling of familiarity—that everything being sensed seems to have happened previously—(the *déjà vu* phenomenon). Often the same hallucination happens again and again, and in such cases the neuro-surgeon can often reproduce the phenomenon by stimulating electrically a sensitive area in the temporal lobe under local anaesthetic; this result is not achieved by stimulating a normal brain.

In these cases, it seems that a *general* recalling system is activated, which can involve the memory mechanisms related to any of the special senses. This general recalling system is probably activated via a part of the brain known as the limbic system (which is discussed in the next chapter), a large part of which (the hippocampus) lies deep in the temporal lobe.

Dreams

Dreaming arises from false activity of the memory and thought systems when the brain is not fully alert and normal. This most obviously occurs when we are asleep. Dreams are known to occur during a particular phase of light sleep. The duration of a dream is very short, and yet the dream often seems to have lasted for a very long time. This loss of a sense of time is presumably due to the 'timing' mechanism of the brain being inactive during sleep. Dreams seem to be made up more of the visual than any other sense. This corresponds with the dominant position of the vision mechanism in our brains.

In retrospect an isolated dream can often be correlated with some experience or thought which occurred the evening before the dream, this being the stimulus that opens up a cache of related memories. But for some people dreams tend repeatedly to re-awaken unwanted memories. The most common example of this type of phenomenon is probably the recurring nightmares experienced by children. My grandchildren tell me that they can prevent this type of nightmare by thinking very hard about the subject of the nightmare before going to sleep.

The investigation of physiological links between types of dream and brain activity is obviously a very complex matter, though it is known that damage to certain parts of the brain completely prevents dreaming. In the next chapter I shall discuss in more detail the memory mechanism whose disturbance brings about dreams and hallucinations.

8

Memory and thought

To exist as 'normal' individuals within the boundaries of accepted social behaviour, we must have brains which are able to perform certain basic tasks. Among these tasks perhaps the most vital are the maintenance of a reasonably reliable memory and the undertaking of (at least) elementary thought processes. For these we must be able to recall both remote and recent events, and arrange them in chronological order.

It is now known that the memory and thought processes of the brain are undertaken mainly by two great systems—the cortex and thalamus form one system, and a region known as the limbic system forms the other. The workings of these two systems are irrevocably intertwined, but this chapter attempts to explain what we do know about their separate functions.

As usual, we learn most about a system and its requirements by observing its failures, and for this reason I shall describe three commonly observed types of memory failure, concluding appropriately with that inevitable failure caused by the effects of old age.

The role of the cortex in thinking

In the past, the enormous development of the cortex of the cerebral hemispheres led man to believe that it controlled all the processes of thought, memory, and learning; however, the cortex is in fact a development of the thalamus (see Fig. 6, p. 22), and is useless without full support from the thalamus. There are very powerful communicating pathways between all parts of the cortex on both sides, and everything that arrives at the cortical receiving areas is likely to travel widely throughout many areas of the brain.

It seems that cortical activity, especially in man, is more concerned with the detailed analysis of arriving information than with the basic needs—of action for survival and so on—yet, at maturity, the basic needs have come to be controlled by cortical analysis. This control of emotions and behaviour is not inborn but must be learnt during childhood.

The analysis of incoming information involves, for example, the selection of items to be stored for future use and the correlation and insertion of these items in their correct context, with previously stored items. The processes of thinking involve the recalling of innumerable sequences of these items one by one, plus the ability to extract individual items from many different sequences, to form other sequences.

This cortex, with its thalamic connections and its interplay between one cortical area and another, seems to be wonderfully self-sufficient for many purposes, but in fact the system seems to be quite useless without the driving forces and controls of the 'limbic system'.

The limbic system

The limbic system incorporates several collections of special types of neurone which are situated in the middle of both cerebral hemispheres close to the thalamus (see Fig. 19). These groups of cells are in close connection with each other and literally make rings round the thalamus; they are thus called the 'limbic circuits'. Each of these little 'organs' in the brain seems to act as a link between the cerebral hemispheres, or one part of the cerebral hemispheres, and primitive structures in the sub-thalamic areas.

The largest of these important circuit structures is the hippocampus; there is one hippocampus in each temporal lobe. If this structure is destroyed on both sides virtually all power of thinking is lost. The hippocampus seems specially

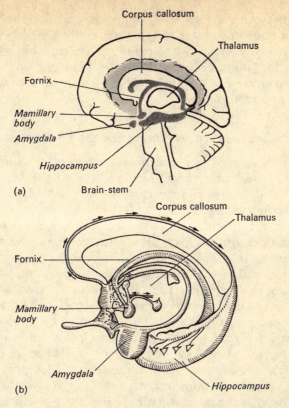

Fig. 19. The limbic system. The brain seems to incorporate at least three powerful neuronal systems which appear to be semi-independent in one sense, but which are entirely dependent on each other. Little is known about how they operate. First there is the alerting system—the reticular formation—in the brain-stem which controls many basic bodily functions, and which is quite essential for survival. Then there are the very extensive cortico-thalamic mechanisms which deal with the most complex aspects of brain activity. Between these two systems is the somewhat mysterious limbic system. The position of these *neuronal systems* in relation to the whole brain is shown in (a). (b) is an enlargement of the central part of (a). The limbic system consists of groups of cells deep in each cerebral hemisphere which communicate with each other around the region of the thalamus. The most complex activities of memory and thinking can not operate without a healthy limbic system.

concerned with the parietal, temporal, and occipital areas of the brain, where new information arrives; for when it is destroyed, the memory of current events can be held for only a few minutes and this renders thought impossible, though remote events can be spoken about in a vague and inconsequential manner.

Co-operation between the cortex and the limbic system

Just as the cortex and thalamus seem to be self-sufficient, so would the limbic system seem to have all that is needed for survival; but in fact the cortical and the limbic systems are interdependent.

The great difficulty is to understand how these powerful organizations control each other, for they have remakably few direct lines of contact. Both systems, however, have very powerful communications with the brain-stem which seems to have considerable influence over brain activity. Also, they both communicate extensively with the thalamus and so can control each other in an indirect way.

This interdependence may be most easily studied in its effect on the visual system of the brain. When visual information reaches the cortex of the occipital lobes from the eyes, if there is nothing unusual about it very little seems to happen, and the information fades away as more information arrives. However, if, on being analysed by the cortex, the visual signals are unusual or of interest, the brain is alerted (to a varying extent) by messages from the cortex to the brain-stem alerting system, and both the cortex and the limbic system are in some way thrown into vigorous activity in order to assess as fully as possible the significance of this visual pattern. For example, a man walking in a busy street with his mind on some problem does not consciously see all the people, buildings, and traffic around him. But if a fire-engine roars down the street towards him his brain systems are alerted and he is jerked out of his reverie.

The formation of a memory

While the brain is under the effect of the alerting system, innumerable repetitions of the visual pattern are made and the cortical activity results in a memory being formed. The main structure of the visual memory seems to be formed in or near to the occipital lobes where the messages arrive, but whether the experience develops into a 'permanent' memory or not seems to depend largely on the amount of encouragement from the limbic system. Indeed if the limbic system is out of action owing to disease or injury, no new memories are ever formed.

It seems that the limbic system is not required for instant repetition, which can hardly be classed as a memory. A colleague of mine had a loudly ticking clock in his laboratory, but he never 'heard' the ticking of the clock unless it suddenly stopped. When it stopped, his brain was suddenly alerted, and he could quite clearly remember hearing the last three ticks. Many people may have had a related experience. In a similar way, if we are suddenly awakened from sleep by a noise we may often be able to remember the sound.

The validity of the argument that the limbic system is not required for these responses can be demonstrated by studying sufferers of Korsakoff's syndrome (which is described on p. 101), a complaint in which the limbic system is totally out of action. The sufferers in this case are able to respond verbally to questions and repeat a number if they do so immediately, although they cannot produce the thought processes which require a more permanent memory of the near past.

The process of thought

It seems that the limbic system provokes thought processes not only by encouraging the original visual pattern to be reactivated over and over again but also by encouraging the recall of similar related experiences in the past. In this way it seems to initiate the early processes of thought.

It does not follow from the extraordinary powers of the

limbic system that the stores of past information are *in* the limbic system itself. The mechanisms are activated throughout the general cortical and thalamic areas of the cerebral hemispheres. Only the cortical mechanisms have the complex organization required to discriminate which details of, say, visual information are to be specially studied. So the cortex must guide or train the limbic system to drive the cortex—in a pattern which the cortex itself must to a large extent determine.

Suppose, for example, that we go to sleep with a problem on our minds. The analysis of the words, emotions, and problems can be effected only by complex cortical activity, but in some way it seems that the intense concentration and interest aroused activates the limbic system to 'drive' the cortical circuits to be active during the hours of sleep, and this may have the following effects.

1. On waking our first thoughts are still of the same subject.
2. Our unsolved problems of yesterday may seem quite easy to deal with.
3. The clarification of yesterday's problems is associated with the recall of some related events or thoughts which were not accessible yesterday.
4. If we dream before waking, it is very probable that some link can be detected between the dream and the events in our thoughts before sleep. Dreams, like hallucinations, seem to be caused by uncontrolled activity of the recalling systems.

The way in which the limbic system can concentrate on one problem in this way suggests that in some parts of it, perhaps in the hippocampus, there must be a specific link with one area of cortex. Almost every aspect of brain activity seems to depend on two-way connections. The hippocampus is enormously developed in man and seems to me to be big enough to have highly localized areas each with special concern for one small area of cortex. Without some very localized point-to-point contact, it is difficult to see how a very technical problem can be picked out for special action during the hours of sleep. However, I know of no anatomical evidence to support this view.

The defective memory

Korsakoff's syndrome

Once again, we can learn much about how the brain works from the symptoms when one of the systems fails. There is a well-known type of memory failure called 'Korsakoff's syndrome', which occurs when the limbic system is put out of action by disease or injury. This disastrous disability was at one time thought to be specially associated with alcoholic insanity but is now known to be due mainly to a severe lack of vitamin B_1 (see p. 99). One link in the limbic circuits evidently depends so much on this vitamin that it disintegrates when deprived of it. Apparently the block in this one small area puts most of the limbic system out of action.

The main feature of Korsakoff's syndrome is often described as a complete failure of recent memory, but in fact it is more accurate to describe it as a complete inability to form new memories. The patient has no knowledge of what happened five minutes ago, so that sequential thought disappears. This produces a hopeless state of confusion, for purposeful thought is impossible and so all initiative is lost. The result is not apparently upsetting to the victim, for the processes which would make him aware of his predicament have also been lost.

An elderly woman, after becoming over-tired, suddenly had a rare variety of 'stroke' which destroyed a vital part of her limbic system. This happened while she was preparing to drive her car, and she was found two hours later sitting in her car doing nothing. Her friend encouraged her to get out of the car, which she did without difficulty, and to walk to the house. She could talk, see, and walk quite well, but from then on she had to be cared for by others. She had been a good cellist, but now she could play only a scale. Sometimes she would disappear for a long walk and be brought back by the police as she knew neither where she was going nor how to return, and soon she could only be looked after in a psychiatric hospital. There she was often visited by her friends; she recognized old friends and could speak of events long past. However, when one of her visiting friends said, 'You do like to see us, don't you?' she replied, 'Haven't I been smiling all the time?'. Later the confusion became worse and she could no longer recognize her friends.

Why the brain needs an uninterrupted blood-supply

In recent years, the term 'transient amnesic episode' has been used to describe a quite startling disorder in which for a period of a few hours the subject develops a Korsakoff syndrome, but then returns to complete normality. This is now thought to be due to a passing interference with the blood-supply to a part of the limbic system, probably the hippocampus.

The blood-supply to most of the hippocampus and to most of the brain-stem reaches the brain via the two vertebral arteries in the neck which pass up towards the skull through small apertures in each neck vertebra. These apertures lie very near to the small joints which are affected by arthritis in most old people. The inflammation round the joints may actually press on the vertebral arteries, squashing the artery quite severely when certain neck movements are made. This can cause a blood clot which blocks circulation to the brain-stem. In this situation, exaggerated neck movements, certain postures, or manipulation of the neck become dangerous, for there is no way of knowing which posture might be doing harm. It is much safer to allow an elderly arthritic neck to become rather stiff, in as comfortable a position as possible.

Because of their connection with the blood-supply of the hippocampus, transient amnesic episodes may follow from such incautious movements as hyper-extension of the neck for long periods, which may occur in a dentist's chair, at the hairdresser, wearing bifocal glasses, decorating the ceiling of a room, swimming breast-stroke, looking upwards, for example at mountains or at a lecture theatre screen, picking fruit, or pruning trees. Turning movements of the neck can also cause trouble if they are exaggerated, as they may be while driving a car, conducting a meeting, or working in awkward corners.

Transient amnesic episodes are only one among several well-known effects of minute strokes caused by the blocking of small brain arteries in the brain-stem. When this effect was first recognized, many neurologists noticed that it was liable to affect elderly men swimming in the sea, and I would once again blame hyper-extension of the neck while swimming breast-stroke for this hazard.

Another example is of a man of about fifty who was standing on a ladder picking apples when the amnesic episode began. In retrospect, the first evidence that this had happened was when he shouted, 'Who brought that wheelbarrow here?' and the answer was, 'Don't be silly, you've just put it there yourself!' He continued to pick the crop for several hours without anyone realizing that anything was wrong but, in the evening, when he was due to help his wife prepare for some visitors who were coming for dinner, he could do nothing to help and his wife realized that he must be ill. Later in the same evening, after dinner, he quite suddenly came to himself and asked what they had been doing. He had a permanent loss of memory for all that had happened since breakfast-time.

A remarkable report appeared in 1969 from two Swiss doctors who had actually succeeded in studying fourteen patients with this transient episode *during* the amnesic period—an amazing achievement. (Perhaps this syndrome is common in Switzerland where people often look up at the mountains!) They reported that during the amnesic period they were able to converse with the patients and found that they could speak only of things that had happened some years previously—as occurs in the fully developed Korsakoff syndrome—but that on recovering after a few hours, the patients seemed to remember everything up to the onset of the episode.

A similar sequence of recovery sometimes emerges after concussion sustained from a head injury, and this sudden jump from retrograde amnesia to normality is an extremely significant feature which must be taken into account in any plausible explanation of the memory mechanism.

The effects of old age

It is well known that as we get older the learning of new material becomes more difficult, and many memories either seem to disappear or cannot be recalled. Current impressions cease to be automatically stored for future use, a diary of appointments becomes more necessary, and we have to go back to make quite sure that we did in fact lock a door or switch off a light.

Because current events are no longer automatically stored for future use, there is a tendency to talk repeatedly of events of long ago, and old memories seem to predominate. There are various possible explanations for the relative strength of old memories. It is possible that early memories, often being of relatively isolated episodes, have not been obscured by many similar experiences. As age advances all new experiences become more complex from the remembering point of view, since every experience has to be correlated and fitted into existing memories. As these existing memories become more numerous, the process of remembering becomes ever more complex.

A memory trace presumably depends on a vast system of modified interneuronal patterns. This is not a static arrangement. Neurones have a habit of discharging spontaneously, and it seems likely that by this means the special patterns of a memory may be maintained or even strengthened with the passage of time. And, of course, it should be realized that the mechanism of forming a new memory must be inherently more complex than recalling an old one, and that as age advances the more complex of the procedures is likely to fail first.

9

Memory chemistry

The brain is a very active organ, and accounts for as much as ten per cent of the total energy expenditure and twenty-five per cent of the total oxygen consumption of the whole body at rest.

Like the rest of the body, the brain obtains its chemical energy by the oxidation of foodstuffs. The primary energy source used by the central nervous system is carbohydrate in the form of the sugar glucose, and in this it differs from other tissues, which are able to use fats and, to a lesser extent, protein. The reason for this is the so-called 'blood–brain barrier' which restricts the entry of many substances. This barrier is a way of protecting the brain against adverse conditions which may prevail in the rest of the body. Unlike organs such as the liver, the brain has little capacity for storage of carbohydrates or fats and, consequently, is dependent on a constant blood-borne supply of glucose and oxygen. If for any reason (such as in a diabetic's insulin coma) this supply is suddenly reduced, unconsciousness results, and if the supply is not restored within minutes irreversible brain damage will occur.

This enormous expenditure of energy by brain cells shows that a vast amount of metabolic activity takes place continually within all parts of the central nervous system. Metabolism is the term used for chemical processes whereby a living thing is maintained and energy derived from the breakdown of foodstuffs is made available for various forms of work.

The brain is composed mainly of two different cell types

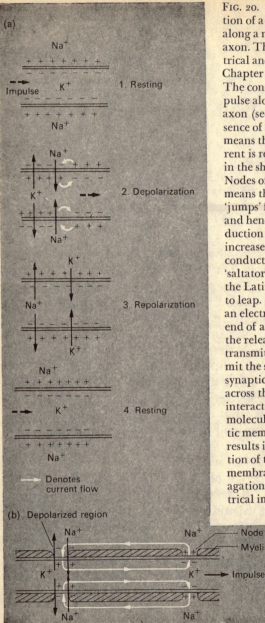

(a)

Na$^+$

+ + + + + + +

Impulse K$^+$ 1. Resting

+ + + + + + +

Na$^+$

Na$^+$

K$^+$ 2. Depolarization

Na$^+$

K$^+$

Na$^+$ 3. Repolarization

K$^+$

Na$^+$

+ + + + + + +

K$^+$ 4. Resting

+ + + + + + +

Na$^+$

→ Denotes
current flow

(b) Depolarized region

Na$^+$ Na$^+$ Node of Ranvier

Myelin sheath

K$^+$ K$^+$ → Impulse

Na$^+$ Na$^+$

Fig. 20. (a) The conduction of a nerve impulse along a non-myelinated axon. This process is electrical and is described in Chapter 10—(p. 135). (b) The conduction of an impulse along a myelinated axon (see p. 110). The presence of a myelin sheath means that the flow of current is restricted to breaks in the sheath known as Nodes of Ranvier. This means that the impulse 'jumps' from node to node and hence the speed of conduction is considerably increased. This type of conduction is known as 'saltatory conduction' from the Latin *saltare*, meaning to leap. (c) The arrival of an electrical signal at the end of an axon results in the release of chemical transmitters which transmit the signal to the post-synaptic cell by diffusing across the synaptic cleft and interacting with a receptor molecule in the postsynaptic membrane (d). This results in the depolarization of the postsynaptic membrane and the propagation of another electrical impulse.

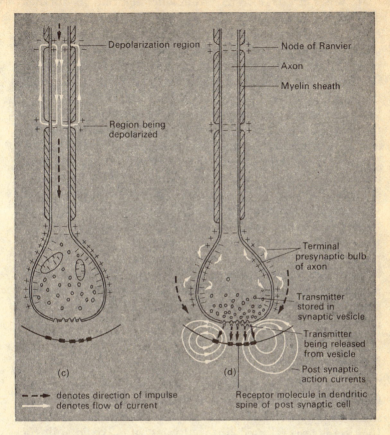

(c)

(d)

Depolarization region

Region being depolarized

Node of Ranvier

Axon

Myelin sheath

Terminal presynaptic bulb of axon

Transmitter stored in synaptic vesicle

Transmitter being released from vesicle

Post synaptic action currents

- - - → denotes direction of impulse
→ denotes flow of current

Receptor molecule in dendritic spine of post synaptic cell

—nerve cells (neurones) and 'glia'—which differ greatly in their properties.

Neurones

As we have seen in Chapter 1, neurones are cells that are specially adapted for the carrying of nerve impulses. Since this process requires a great deal of energy it is not surprising to find that the neurones have a high metabolic rate; they use between ten and a hundred times more oxygen than the glia, and their rate of protein synthesis is also substantially higher.

Impulses are transferred from one neurone to another at synapses (see Fig. 20). The synapse is where one neurone comes into functional contact with another, but there is no direct contact between one neurone and the next. The mechanism by which nerve impulses spread across the synapses in the human brain is believed to be exclusively chemical, although there are a few interesting cases in some animals where transmission is known to be electrical, for example, in the nerve cord of earthworms and crayfish and in the brain of a goldfish. When an impulse reaches the end of the axon it causes release of a chemical neuro-transmitter (see below) which diffuses rapidly across the synaptic cleft and excites the cell on the other side of the synapse (the postsynaptic cell). The neurotransmitter is then quickly destroyed by an enzyme to prevent its continued action. (Enzymes are 'catalysts' responsible for regulating the chemical reactions in the cell; all enzymes are proteins.) In addition to these synapses which transmit activity there are also inhibitory synapses, where the released neurotransmitter inhibits activity in the postsynaptic cell.

Neurotransmitters

There is still a great deal to be learnt about neurotransmitters. What we do know is that they are contained in small bags ('synaptic vesicles', see Fig. 20) at the nerve endings and are released in multiples of a basic unit (a 'quantum'). They are released by nervous stimulation and, when applied to the next cell, on the 'far' side of the synapse, reproduce the effect of stimulating the cell on the 'near' side.

A number of different substances seem to act as transmitters in the nervous system. The best-known of these are acetylcholine and noradrenaline, which is similar to adrenaline. Nerve fibres containing the former are termed 'cholinergic', and those containing the latter 'noradrenergic'.

Acetylcholine is present in high concentrations in the thalamus, hippocampus, and cerebral cortex, and cholinergic neurones are believed to be of importance in some of the connections of specific sensory pathways. Noradrenaline is found in the brain-stem and hypothalamus (see Fig. 3; p. 5). There is also evidence for the existence of two other neurotransmitters, called 5-hydroxytryptamine (5-HT) and dopamine (both of which have molecules similar to noradrenaline; molecules of this family are termed 'biogenic amines').

All these neurotransmitters are thought to be excitatory (with the exception of acetylcholine which may be both excitatory and inhibitory depending on where it is released). There are also two other molecules, γ-amino butyric acid (GABA) and glycine (of the group called amino acids), which appear to be inhibitory neurotransmitters in the cortex and spinal cord respectively.

Studies on the biochemistry of these intriguing substances are especially important since it is becoming increasingly apparent that disorders in the metabolism of neurotransmitters play a large part in certain mental illnesses. For instance, schizophrenia and depressive illnesses may involve disturbances of the transmitters similar to noradrenaline, neurones containing dopamine may be affected in Parkinson's disease, and malfunctions in the cholinergic and GABA-containing neuronal systems could be involved in epilepsy.

Glia

Glia are generally much smaller cells than neurones and are packed between them. They differ from neurones in that they do not conduct electrical signals or transmit these signals chemically from cell to cell (and hence have no axons or synapses) and, because they can divide, they can recover from injury which neurones cannot do. Their lower metabolic rate has already been mentioned.

Glia are believed to play a nutritive and supportive role and are also important in synthesizing and breaking down the transmitters released by the neurones. It is also possible that they provide chemical and electrical insulation between groups of synapses on the same cell body.

The development of the brain

Neurones and glia differ also in their patterns of development. Brain maturation may be considered to occur in two main stages. In the first stage the neurones are formed. When the adult number of neurones is attained there is no further division of these cells. In man, the adult number of neurones is reached approximately two-thirds of the way through the development of the foetus in pregnancy.

In the second stage there is growth of axons and dendrites, establishment of neural connections, and multiplication of special glial cells which then deposit coats (called 'myelin sheaths') on the nerve fibres to insulate them, very like the insulation on electric cables. This process, called 'myelination', makes nerve-impulse conduction much faster. Myelination only ever occurs during this stage, and once laid down the myelin will remain unchanged throughout life. It is during this period that the white matter (containing mainly nerve fibres) and the grey matter (containing mainly nerve-cell bodies) become distinguishable (see Fig. 5, p. 21).

This second stage, in which brain growth is at its fastest, is sometimes termed the 'growth spurt' and in man lasts from the last two or three months of gestation until two years after birth. By the age of six, the brain has reached ninety-five per cent of its adult size. Man is thus a perinatal ('around birth') developer, and in this he differs from a number of other mammals. For instance, in the guinea-pig the growth spurt occurs entirely in the foetus (prenatal development) and in the rat the growth spurt takes place after birth (postnatal development).

Because the laboratory rat is a postnatal developer biochemists have been able to study in detail the metabolic changes accompanying the growth spurt. During this period the enzymes involved in the manufacture of vital chemicals are more active than in the adult brain. The proliferation of glia is mirrored by an increase in brain DNA. DNA is a giant 'informational' molecule and makes up the hereditary material of genes and chromosomes. Every cell containing DNA in the body has the same quantity of DNA in its nucleus, and hence any increase in the number of cells must involve an increase in DNA.

Any disturbances of metabolism during this vulnerable period of the growth spurt can have very grave and irreversible consequences. In particular, malnutrition produces catastrophic results. We have seen how the brain is dependent on a constant supply of chemical energy. During the growth spurt the demand for energy is at its greatest, and malnutrition will drastically reduce the energy available for the manufacturing processes crucial to the development of the brain. This can result in an irreversible reduction in brain size, the total number of cells, and the degree of myelination. Starvation in adults does not produce the same effect—in fact the adult brain is remarkably resistant to the effects of malnutrition.

In a laboratory experiment a group of rats belonging to a small litter was brought up alongside another group of rats in an artificially enlarged litter, until the time of weaning at twenty-one days. The nutritionally deprived rats of the larger litter had lower body-weight, brain-weight, brain-cell number, and myelination. The difference between litters persisted into adulthood even though all the rats were given as much food as they wanted after twenty-one days. Experiments of this type have yielded information of great relevance to the problems of a world in which over half the human population is undernourished.

DNA, RNA, and what they do

Biochemists have been fascinated by the chemical mechanisms in learning and memory. There has been a long—and continuing—search for the controversial 'memory molecule' that would change when a memory was formed and could possibly be transferred to another animal, which would then have that specific memory. Although a few biochemical hypotheses were put forward earlier, it has been since the

1950s, following the great advances in molecular biology (for instance, the discovery of the structure of DNA by Watson and Crick), that research into the biochemical basis of memory has gained momentum.

The genetic information of living cells is now known to be stored in the form of the nucleic acid called DNA (deoxyribonucleic acid) which is situated in the cell nucleus. The sequence of certain components of the molecule makes up a code or language carried on DNA, called the genetic code. The information stored in the DNA is conveyed to the body of the cell by first 'transcribing' the genetic code into another nucleic acid, 'messenger RNA' (ribonucleic acid), from which the code is 'translated' into protein. The code on the RNA determines the protein's properties and role in the cell.

A possible 'memory molecule'?

The storage of genetic information in an 'informational' giant molecule has been referred to as an example of a biological 'memory', because one cell can divide to reproduce two replicas of itself containing the same information. This process of cell division and replacement takes place continually in all organs and tissues of the body (apart from mature neurones).

The discovery of the mechanism for this genetic type of memory led some biochemists to suggest that the cerebral type of memory might be stored in a similar way. However, since DNA is stable in non-dividing cells and the neurones of the brain do not divide. DNA could be ruled out as a possible 'memory molecule'. RNA or protein appeared to be more likely candidates, since they can be synthesized according to the needs of the cell. (Proteins are made up of units known as amino acids; the ordering of these units gives a mechanism for storing information.)

The brain contains a great deal of RNA. Neurones are among the most active producers of RNA in the body; the glial cells have, on average, much less. The brain also has a very high turnover of protein, which is curious since, unlike some organs, the brain does not secrete protein to another part of the body. The bulk of protein is synthesized in the main cell body of the neurones but can be transported down the axon to the nerve ending. The active RNA and protein metabolism seen in neurones is similar to that seen in rapidly dividing cells but, since neurones do not divide, RNA and protein may have a special functional role in the brain.

In the last decade or so many experiments have been carried out to try and prove that RNA and protein are involved in certain aspects of brain activity. The results are very ambiguous, probably because of the extreme difficulties encountered in designing adequately controlled experiments. However, the bulk of the results point to a connection between the rate of RNA and protein metabolism and the functional state of the nervous tissue, and they show that RNA and protein metabolism must be in some way involved in the fixation of memory.

The effects of submitting a variety of animals to frequent changes of posture and to olfactory, auditory, and visual stimulation have been studied. In most cases the stimulation was followed by an increased metabolism of RNA and protein in the brain cells concerned with receiving these stimuli.

Some especially significant research on mammalian neurones and on the neurones of a sea-slug has shown that the increased RNA in a cell depended on activation via its dendritic synapses, and that the events at the synapse involving the transmitter were responsible for 'triggering off' the change in RNA metabolism in the cell body.

These studies have given convincing evidence of a relationship between nervous activity and RNA metabolism in nervous tissue. This relationship is further supported by a study of the pattern of RNA synthesis in the cortex of a rabbit during sleep, which showed that the pattern of synthesis of RNA was influenced by the state of cortical electrical activity.

Environmental influences on the chemical activity of the brain

A research group at the University of California at Berkeley have done some experiments which may be of great significance. They found that the brains of rats reared in conditions of environmental complexity and constant exposure to stimulation had an increased cortical weight and protein content, and increased activity of enzymes controlling the metabolism of the transmitter acetylcholine, compared with the brains of similar rats kept in isolation in a severely restricted environment and subject to minimal stimulation.

These studies may well throw light on the plight of deprived children who seem to be faced with insuperable difficulties in their education; these matters are considered further in Chapter Eleven.

The chemistry of learning

Those experiments which involve exposure to movement, smell, hearing, or vision are referred to by the scientists concerned as 'exposure to passive stimulation', but attempts have also been made to study the effects of some more purposeful type of stimulation which would be more compatible with the terms 'memory' and 'learning'. However, this distinction is probably misleading, for, as previous chapters have described, the methods of alerting the brain to action are so numerous and variable that they could hardly be divided so crudely.

Research has shown that administration of drugs which inhibit synthesis of RNA and protein in the brain interferes with the ability of animals to learn. There are several controversial reports that drugs which stimulate this synthesis actually enhance learning ability. Evidence is also accumulating that learning results in the synthesis of new RNA and protein in specific brain areas. There are experiments which suggest that some of the proteins involved in these changes are specific to the brain.

However, although these experiments demonstrate fairly convincingly that RNA and protein synthesis are required for learning, they do not provide evidence for a specific memory molecule, and this concept is tending to become discredited. The only experiments which set out to demonstrate directly the existence of such a molecule are the transfer experiments, in which attempts have been made to transfer knowledge by injecting a brain RNA extract from a trained animal to an untrained animal. Positive results have been claimed using both rats and a species of flatworm but the results of such experiments have been widely disputed.

It now appears that the 'transfer factor' is likely to be a contaminant of the RNA extract. One group have actually claimed to have isolated a substance (called 'scotophobin') which could be classed as a memory molecule—a substance which transfers the reaction 'avoidance of the dark' in rats.

There have been attempts to apply this transfer approach to the treatment of prematurely senile patients by giving them massive doses of RNA, without proven success.

Most of these ideas appear unrealistic and theoretically unsound to those who study brain mechanisms, but there is here one point of enormous interest. In man, the RNA content of the brain neurones increases until the age of forty, remains constant for the next two decades, and falls rapidly after the age of sixty. This age-curve is of special interest for it is entirely different from the age-curve for learning ability, which reaches its maximum at about the age of sixteen years, and diminishes steadily thereafter. There is therefore no correlation between the 'amount of learning' and the amount of RNA. But, on the other hand, there may well be a correlation between the amount of brain RNA and the amount of brain activity, for, during adult life, every thought acquires new connections and complexities, while every decision, and every 'amount of learning', requires more time in order to consider the ever-increasing number of factors involved. After the age of sixty, memories begin to disappear and the amount of new learning generally decreases, so that brain activity becomes steadily more restricted, and this might well be reflected in the drop in RNA in the old person's brain.

What is a memory?

Here a warning should be given about the ambiguities of words such as 'memory', 'learning', and 'memory trace'. Each user of such terms has a different idea of what they mean. Thus we know that when neurones in the brain are activated by a sensory input, there ensues a train of events between a vast number of brain cells, which may be followed by some kind of response. If this response, on repetition, becomes established, then this elementary germ of a memory must bring about changes in relation to the cells. It is the precise nature of these changes that we all hope very much to discover some day.

There have been many attempts to invoke separate mechanisms for short-term and long-term memory, but I think that this is better avoided, as the one mechanism merges imperceptibly into the other when we come to study the normal person. As has been emphasized earlier, whether an episode is remembered for a long time, for a short time, or not at all depends on a host of circumstances, none of which can be clearly distinguished.

How do we form a memory?

Many biochemical researches have been directed towards the study of memory. What can be concluded from the welter of experimental facts?

Currently there are two main theories—an *intra*neuronal theory, which suggests that memory is encoded chemically within neurones; and an *inter*neuronal theory which suggests that memory is stored in the form of relationships between large numbers of neurones. There is little evidence to support the first theory, but the second is becoming more widely accepted. The formation of new relationships between neurones implies growth of nerve endings and dendrites to form new synaptic connections. The formation of these new functional structures would require RNA and protein synthesis, and this could explain why changes in RNA and protein synthesis have been shown to occur during learning. Since protein is synthesized largely in the neurone cell body, protein must be newly synthesized and travel from the cell body down the axon to the synapse, within the time required for memory consolidation.

Protein molecules can be synthesized as rapidly as one per second, and some proteins are transported down the axon at rates of several centimetres per day. This means that proteins could reach some nerve endings in the nervous system within minutes. Even with long axons (a few millimetres in length) the protein could reach the nerve endings within a few hours. Thus the interneuronal hypothesis appears to be consistent with our present knowledge about the rate of formation of memory.

Since individual molecules of protein in the brain last only for a few weeks, the proteins involved in maintaining a long-term memory must be constantly renewed. In other words, each neurone must be continually engaged in preserving the current state of its synapses. These chemical researches do provide a revised picture of the method whereby a neuronal sequence in intercommunication can strengthen itself. Thus repetitive activity must be associated with the synthesizing of new protein molecules which are then pushed down the axon to strengthen or enlarge the dendrites of those other cells which have come to accept the pulses arriving via this particular axon.

Clearly the receiving cell must have the power to choose between different pulses arriving from different cells, and this is perhaps the most fascinating problem of all. Perhaps the cell 'prefers' pulses from one particular axon because the properties of the dendrite have been altered in some way by the newly synthesized protein. On the other hand, the intervention of inhibiting enzyme activity from 'downstream' must provide a feed-back which controls the synaptic activity 'up-stream'. Remember that powerful inhibiting systems operate on the brain as a whole in order to allow full attention to be paid to one particular matter.

10

Drugs that act on the brain

For centuries, man has known that extracts from certain plants can produce stimulation, sedation, or even psychological effects alien to his everyday existence. For common examples of substances which produce stimulation and sedation respectively one has to look no further than coffee and alcohol. Plant extracts producing heightened psychological effects were used widely by primitive tribes and ancient civilizations during religious ceremonies.

We are now able to use such substances (known as psychoactive drugs) to treat certain medical and psychiatric disorders, partly because our knowledge of chemistry enables us to extract, identify, and synthesize many of the active ingredients of these plants, and partly because there has been a remarkable increase in the knowledge of brain chemistry over the last twenty years or so. One of the major breakthroughs was the discovery that a number of these drugs altered the metabolism of the brain biogenic amines (which were discussed on p. 109), and in some cases resembled them in chemical structure.

Psychoactive drugs may be considered to fall into two broad categories: substances with a depressant effect and substances with a stimulatory effect.

Depressants

Barbiturates and alcohol

Some of the most well-known depressants of the central

nervous system are the barbiturates. Barbiturates are used as sedatives, sleeping pills, anaesthetics, and anticonvulsants in the control of epilepsy. The way in which barbiturates, such as phenobarbitone and amytal, act on the brain is still not completely understood, although it is believed that they may interfere with the production of chemical energy.

We now consume enormous quantities of barbiturates. This is dramatically illustrated by the fact that in 1968 25 million prescriptions for barbiturates were issued in Great Britain alone. It has even been estimated that every tenth night's sleep in the United Kingdom is induced by sleeping pills. Statistics indicate that a large number of people are psychologically dependent on these drugs, that is, they are unable to live a normal life without them. Dependence is different from addiction. Addiction is a clearly defined clinical state and is characterized by three features: psychological dependence, change in tolerance to the drug (that is, the addict requires more and more of the drug to produce the same effect and eventually is able to tolerate doses which would be fatal if taken by a non-addict), and the occurrence of 'withdrawal symptoms' if the drug is suddenly withheld.

For the true barbiturate addict, barbiturates have a stimulating rather than sedating effect. The withdrawal symptoms, or 'abstinence syndrome' as it is known clinically, include epileptic fits followed by a state in which acute anxiety, disorientation, tremulousness, and visual hallucinations occur.

Alcohol is also a depressant drug and actually suppresses cortical activity, although its effects may appear to us to be excitatory. The reason for this apparent paradox is that the excitatory effects of alcohol are due to depression of inhibitory systems in the higher centres of the brain. The first mental processes to be affected are those that depend on training and self-restraint. Alcohol thus impairs the functions concerned with perception of what is 'good' or 'bad', socially acceptable or socially unacceptable. In effect, alcohol 'dissolves' the conscience, and as a result the drinker of alcohol feels free of his inhibitions. He becomes more confident and vivacious but is prone to emotional outbursts and rapid changes of mood. However, the suppression of cortical activity is related to the alcohol level in the blood, and as this level rises the so-called 'lower' functions become affected. This accounts for the unsteadiness of gait, slurring of speech, and even unconsciousness which are features of the more advanced stages of alcohol intoxication. In extreme cases the activity of the brain area responsible for respiration is affected, and death may result.

Alcohol is, of course, widely used in society to increase relaxation and promote good fellowship in company, and it plays an important part in celebrations of success or in consoling failure. However, alcohol is one of the most abused of all drugs. It has been estimated that the incidence of alcoholism (alcohol addiction) in the United Kingdom is approximately one per cent of the population. It is four times more prevalent in males than in females.

Generally alcoholism develops in three main stages. In the first stage the subject indulges in excessive drinking during which his tolerance for alcohol increases so that he requires more drink to produce the same pleasurable sensations. The next stage is shown by alcoholic amnesia—the drinker has no memory of the hours during which he has been drinking. On wakening in the morning the subject has violent fits of trembling (known as 'the shakes') and a feeling of apprehension. These symptoms can be stopped by taking a drink, but if they are not stopped in this way the DTs (*Delirium tremens*) result. *Delirium tremens* is the withdrawal symptom of alcohol addiction and is characterized by disorientation and terrifying hallucinations.

In past centuries alcohol was used as a crude anaesthetic, for instance during amputation operations after military battles. This brings us to another very important use of depressant drugs.

The relief of pain

Some drugs which depress the central nervous system

are important in medicine for the relief of pain. Such drugs are termed analgesics.

An extract of the seed capsules of the oriental poppy (*Papaver somniferum*) contains a number of potent pain-killers. This extract is opium. The psychological effects of opium were discovered as long ago as 4000 B.C., and there is reference to its actions in writings from the third century B.C. By the seventeenth century the medicinal properties of opium were so well known that one writer of this period could state that 'among the remedies which it has pleased Almighty God to give to man to relieve his sufferings, none is so universal and so efficacious as opium.'

The most important of the score or so of pain-relieving substances in opium (opium alkaloids) is morphine, whose precise mode of action is by no means understood. It is believed to affect the spinal cord, the cerebral cortex, and the limbic system and, in so doing, reduces fear, anxiety, the power of concentration, and any sensations of prolonged pain. This produces a great feeling of contentment and euphoria, which explains why opium has had a long history of abuse. By the eighteenth century opium smoking was so widespread in the Orient that the trade in opium became of major commercial importance. In fact the trade was so remunerative to the merchants that when in 1839 the Chinese Government attempted to reduce their country's opium consumption by confiscating imported opium, the so-called 'Opium wars' broke out and lasted for three years.

The popular picture conjured up by opium abuse is of dingy smokey opium dens full of lethargic orientals. However, opium was also used widely in more 'respectable' circles. A solution of opium in alcohol, known as laudanum, was regarded as a general panacea in the early Victorian era, and was even used to quieten babies. The Victorian novelist Wilkie Collins was addicted to laudanum, and centred the plot of his novel *The Moonstone* around its effects. Opium and its derivatives were freely available in Britain until as late as 1920, when the Dangerous Drugs Act was introduced.

Morphine was isolated from opium in 1803, and by the

mid-nineteenth century pure morphine and other extracted opium alkaloids were used medicinally. Although a most potent pain-killer, morphine is addictive, and this makes it dangerous. Its chemical actions are still under investigation. It is known to affect the release of the transmitters acetylcholine and noradrenaline and to block certain actions of 5-HT (these transmitters are described on p. 109) but the relevance of these effects to its pain-killing action are not yet known. Morphine not only increases the pain threshold (that is, it reduces the sensation of pain) but, more importantly, actually prevents the pain sensation from evoking fear and suffering.

Addiction to the products of opium, or 'narcotics', has become a pressing social problem which can be traced back to the general availability of opium fifty years ago. And the invention of the hypodermic needle in 1853 also helped to increase the use of these drugs. At first it was hoped that if the drugs were not ingested they would not be addictive, but unfortunately the reverse turned out to be the case. In America the abuse of opium products was increased by the influx of opium-smoking Chinese labourers and also by the widespread use of morphine by wounded soldiers during the Civil War.

In 1896 a compound chemically related to morphine, known as heroin (diacetyl morphine), was introduced. Heroin is an even more potent pain-killer than morphine, but the risk of early addiction is even higher. Rather curiously it was regarded as non-addictive until 1915. Heroin addiction has increased dramatically in recent years. There are now over 400 times more known heroin addicts in the world than there were twenty years ago.

At first the morphine or heroin user develops increased tolerance to the drug and requires larger and larger doses to get a 'kick'. Addiction can occur even after a mere two or three days of drug use and is indicated by the appearance of withdrawal symptoms if doses are discontinued. These symptoms are similar for both morphine and heroin and are prolonged, unpleasant, and dangerous. Within a few hours of withdrawal the addict becomes very active and irritable. He perspires heavily, his eyes water, and he yawns frequently. The yawning can be so violent that jaw dislocation results. These symptoms reach a peak after two or three days and the addict becomes so restless that he paces up and down like a caged animal. At this time there is loss of appetite, severe sneezing, nausea, diarrhoea, and vomiting. The heart-rate and blood-pressure increase, and the body alternates between flushing and excessive sweating and periods of chilliness and goose-pimples. The goose-flesh is so prominent that the skin resembles that of a plucked turkey; hence the expression 'cold turkey' used to describe sudden withdrawal from these drugs. Painful muscular cramps occur and muscle spasms and kicking movements are common. These symptoms are indicative of increased excitability in the central nervous system. Sometimes this excitability is increased to the extent that sexual orgasm occurs. After this period the symptoms decline in severity over the next week but the addict remains anxious, extremely weak, and depressed. His appetite remains poor and he suffers from insomnia. Only after two or three months can he be said to have returned to even moderate health.

In view of the dangers of addiction, narcotic analgesics are medically used only in cases of extreme pain and are withdrawn as soon as possible. However, they are of immense value in the treatment of pain in terminal illnesses like cancer, where the risk of addiction is a secondary consideration. For the relief of pain of slight to moderate intensity, less powerful but non-addictive drugs are used.

The class of drug most widely used for the relief of mild pain is the salicylates, of which aspirin (acetylsalicylic acid) is the best-known example. Salicylates occur naturally in willow bark, but all the drugs used today are produced by chemical synthesis. Aspirin was first synthesized in 1899. It selectively depresses the central nervous system but probably not the cerebral cortex; this is concluded from the fact that analgesic doses sufficient to stop pain do not cause mental disturbances. Since most pain impulses arrive at the thalamus, aspirin is thought to act by blocking the pain centres in this area. Aspirin also affects the hypothalamus—the brain area which controls body temperature and which is the 'thermostat' of the body. Aspirin has the effect of 're-setting' the thermostat for normal temperature and is consequently used for bringing down the temperature in feverish patients. A third action of aspirin is as an anti-inflammatory agent, and it is used frequently for the alleviation of rheumatic conditions.

In high doses aspirin has toxic effects both on the stomach (where it can cause ulcers) and on the brain. It can cause confusion, dizziness, delirium, stupor, and coma. Aspirin poisoning can also produce deafness to high tones and ringing in the ears due to an increase in pressure in the inner ear.

Aspirin is usually used combined with other analgesics, for example, codeine (methyl morphine) and phenacetin, to provide more effective pain relief. Codeine is chemically very similar to morphine but, to produce the same effect as 10 mg of morphine, 120 mg of codeine is required. With codeine, however, there is far less risk of addiction: 32 mg of codeine will produce the same analgesic effect as 600 mg of aspirin. In addition to raising the pain threshold, codeine, like morphine, tends to dissociate the pain sensation from suffering, that is, it enables the patient to tolerate the pain more readily. Codeine is especially useful as an 'antitussive', that is, a substance that reduces coughing.

Tranquillizers

The so-called 'major tranquillizers' or 'neuroleptics' are drugs which are used for treating psychoses and have the effect of producing sedation without causing sleep. In India the Rauwolfia alkaloids were used for centuries for treating insanity. In 1952 the active ingredient 'reserpine' was isolated from the root of the shrub *Rauwolfia serpentine* and was found to have neuroleptic properties. Reserpine has the effect of depleting brain biogenic amines by blocking the uptake of the amines, after their synthesis, into their storage sites in the neurone. This results in newly formed amines being rapidly broken down by the enzyme monoamine oxidase (MAO), and thus interference with transmission. It is thought that the tranquillizing effect of reserpine is due to the reduction in brain amine levels.

Reserpine, although of great theoretical interest, has the disadvantage that it can cause severe mental depression. In some cases this is so severe that it can lead to suicide. It has been largely superseded by two other groups of major tranquillizers—the phenothiazines and the butyrophenones. The best-known drugs in these groups are chlorpromazine and haloperidol. The former is especially widely used to control such conditions as mania and schizophrenia. Their action is not fully understood, but there is evidence that they interfere with the transmitter dopamine.

The minor tranquillizers (known as 'anxiolytic sedatives') are not effective in treating psychoses but are widely used in controlling the stages of anxiety and agitation that seem to be affecting more and more people in the modern world. The well-known drugs chlordiazepoxide (librium), diazepam (valium), and mogadon come into this category. Librium and valium reduce the spontaneous activity in the hippocampus and the arousal response to stimulation of the brainstem. Librium and valium have the reputation of being very safe, and cases of poisoning with these drugs are indeed rare. However, excessive use can lead to physical dependence and withdrawal symptoms if the drug is stopped. These symptoms include seizures, depression, agitation, insomnia, and lack of appetite. Librium, if taken in toxic doses, can produce nausea, skin rash, impairment of sexual function, vertigo, and menstrual irregularities.

Antidepressants

In contrast to the action of major tranquillizers, drugs that have an antidepressant action have been shown to increase brain amine levels either by inhibiting the enzyme that breaks them down (monoamine oxidase, MAO) or by blocking the reception of amines by the axon terminal after transmission. Drugs that act in the former manner are called MAO inhibitors. Drugs that block uptake are the tricyclic antidepressants (so called because of their chemical structure). The opposing action of tranquillizers and antidepressants on the brain biogenic amines suggests that depression may be associated with an absolute or relative deficiency of these amines, whereas elation may be associated with an excess of them. This amine hypothesis to explain 'affective disorders' was put forward in the 1950s, but subsequent research has indicated that the situation is really far more complicated. 'Affective disorders' is the name given to mental illnesses in which alteration of mood is a major symptom, for example, manic depressive illness.

Stimulants

In addition to the antidepressants there is a group of widely known substances which act as direct stimulants of the central nervous system.

Amphetamine and cocaine

The Chinese used the herb 'ma-huang' for thousands of years. During the last century its active ingredient, ephedrine, was isolated, and later a similar substance, amphetamine, was synthesized. This drug produces a feeling of wakefulness, alertness, and elation, and enables the more rapid performance of tasks such as mental arithmetic. Amphetamine's chemical structure is similar to that of noradrenaline, and it is possible that it enhances the action of brain noradrenaline.

Amphetamines are used to treat mild depressive conditions and, because they reduce the appetite as well as increasing physical activity, are sometimes used for treating obesity.

A number of social factors have led to misuse of amphetamines—for instance, their use by students for the purpose of staying awake at night to revise for exams or by lorry drivers to prevent themselves from falling asleep during long journeys. The abuse of amphetamine and related drugs may take the form of consumption of 'pep pills' or, more seriously, the intravenous injection of the drug. When used intravenously amphetamine is known as 'speed'. On injection the user experiences an intensely pleasurable sensation and has a sense of enhanced physical strength and mental and sexual powers. He has no need for sleep nor food. The effect of amphetamine is of short duration and is followed by a period of depression, lassitude, and fatigue.

Perpetual users of the drug may become addicted to it, but the dependence is primarily emotional rather than physical. Although there are no withdrawal symptoms from amphetamine-like drugs apart from a craving for the drug, there is a serious risk of poisoning. As the user becomes tolerant to the drug he will require greater and more frequent doses, and toxic symptoms can appear. These include grinding of the teeth, repetitive behaviour, and eventually hallucinations and symptoms akin to those of schizophrenia. In some cases the user becomes homicidal: a world-wide survey undertaken in 1968 showed that, of all the admissions into psychiatric units, jails, and remand homes, between eight and eighteen per cent showed evidence of having taken amphetamine.

Devotees of Sherlock Holmes will be aware that the drug cocaine also stimulates the cerebral cortex and facilitates mental activity. Cocaine is often referred to as a narcotic, but from the pharmacological point of view it closely resembles amphetamine; strictly, the term 'narcotic' should only be used to describe drugs similar to morphine. The toxic effects of cocaine are similar to those of amphetamine but appear more rapidly. From the clinical point of view the most important action of cocaine is its ability to block the conduction of impulses along certain nerves. This makes it a very effective local anaesthetic since, when applied to a particular area, it will prevent the impulses associated with pain from being conducted to the brain. It is no longer used as such because it is so addictive.

Tea, coffee, and cocoa

Perhaps the most familiar and widely used stimulants of

the central nervous system are caffeine, theophylline, and theobromine. Coffee contains caffeine, tea contains caffeine and theophylline, and cocoa contains caffeine and theobromine. Caffeine is also present in some soft drinks, notably the cola-flavoured ones.

The strongest stimulant of the three is caffeine, and the amount contained in one or two cups of coffee is enough to stimulate mental activity and reduce fatigue and drowsiness. The way in which these stimulants act is unknown, but there is evidence that they stimulate energy production in the body.

Tea and coffee are so established as staple items in our way of life that it is difficult to think of them as 'drugs'. However, it is amusing to find that in the last century pharmacological experts issued dire warnings on the effects of excessive tea and coffee consumption. Tea was described as 'especially efficient in producing nightmares with hallucinations which may be alarming in their intensity' and was said to 'produce a strange and extreme degree of physical depression and make the speech become weak and vague'. The author concluded by stating that 'by miseries such as these the best years of life may be spoilt.' The effects of coffee were described in equally alarming terms. In contrast, the same authorities could state that 'opium is used rightly or wrongly in many oriental countries, not as an idle or vicious indulgence but as a reasonable aid in the work of life.' These quotations provide a salutary reminder of how society's reactions to different drugs can change over a relatively short period.

Caffeine has indeed some toxic effects and can cause insomnia, restlessness, ringing in the ears, and increased heart-rate and respiration-rate. Convulsions and death can occur after ingestion of ten grams of caffeine, but to achieve this a coffee drinker would have to consume approximately eighty cups in quick succession. Medicinally, caffeine is used for treating cases of poisoning by depressant drugs like morphine.

It is interesting that in primates, including man, there is a substance called uric acid in the blood which has a very similar chemical structure to caffeine (see Fig. 21). This substance is produced by breaking down the body's nucleic acids. It is very insoluble, and when it comes out of solution causes gout. In most animals there is an enzyme which breaks down uric acid but this is absent in man and the primates.

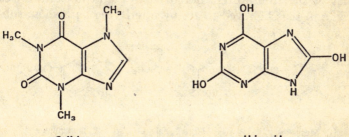

Caffeine   Uric acid

FIG. 21. The chemical structure of uric acid is similar to that of caffeine.

In 1955 Orowan suggested that uric acid, like caffeine, might have a stimulating action on the central nervous system and thus by losing, during the course of evolution, the enzyme responsible for its breakdown, the primates carry a central nervous system stimulant in their blood. He further suggested that this may be one of the factors contributing to the superior intellect of primates. Although this idea may seem rather far-fetched, there had been some rather interesting evidence collected to support it. For instance, in independent surveys carried out on business executives in Edinburgh and on American university professors, it was found that human characteristics such as 'drive', 'leadership', and 'achievement' were associated with high uric acid levels in the blood. There is also some evidence that levels of uric acid change in manic depressive illness and that in families with a history of manic depressive illness there is also a history of gout.

Hallucinogens

Drugs that produce abnormal phenomena in the cognitive

and perceptual areas of the brain are known as 'psychodysleptics' or, more commonly, hallucinogens and psychedelics.

At the turn of the century it was found that an extract of the cactus *Lophophora williamsi* had hallucinogenic effects. The substance found to be responsible for these effects was mescaline. Its chemical structure is remarkably similar to that of the transmitters noradrenaline and dopamine (see Fig. 22). It is believed to act by interfering with those sub-

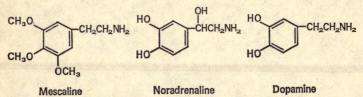

Mescaline   Noradrenaline   Dopamine

FIG. 22. Mescaline (an extract from a cactus) is in structure remarkably similar to noradrenaline and dopamine.

stances in the brain, although as yet the mechanisms involved are not really understood.

Likewise, the action of lysergic acid diethylamide (LSD) is obscure, although there is evidence to suggest that it interferes with the transmitters noradrenaline and serotonin in the brain. LSD is a derivative of lysergic acid which occurs in ergot-producing fungi. LSD was first synthesized in 1943 by Hoffman who discovered its hallucinatory effects when he accidentally inhaled the dust.

He described his experience in the following terms. 'I was seized by a peculiar sensation of vertigo and restlessness. Objects, as well as the shape of my associates in the laboratory, appeared to undergo optical changes. I was unable to concentrate on my work. In a dream-like state I left for home where an irresistible urge to lie down overcame me. I drew the curtains and immediately fell into a peculiar state similar to drunkenness, characterized by an exaggerated imagination. With my eyes closed, fantastic pictures of extraordinary plasticity and intensive colour seemed to surge towards me. After two hours this state gradually wore off.'

The response of subjects to LSD can vary considerably. In some the user may experience great lucidity of thought, enhanced awareness of his surroundings, and an ecstatic transcendental experience. On the other hand, a user may become confused and experience fear and panic with complete loss of emotional control. This is commonly known as a 'bad trip'.

LSD is rapidly absorbed after oral administration and is distributed widely throughout the body. It is concentrated in the liver where it is chemically modified and is excreted in a different form.

Although its most significant effect is on the brain, little LSD is found there after a dose. In fact LSD is the most potent hallucinogen known and is effective in remarkably low doses. In susceptible individuals only twenty or thirty micrograms are required to produce an effect.

Although there are uses for LSD in psychiatry, its use in an uncontrolled manner without proper medical supervision is to be deplored. Many complications and adverse reactions can occur from its misuse. An individual in the midst of a 'good trip' may indulge in dangerous activities such as attempting to fly out of a high window. On the other hand, an individual suffering a 'bad trip' may become homicidal and act in a manner that puts other members of society in danger. He may also be plunged into a state of such despair that suicide is attempted. In addition to anxiety, panic, and violent paranoia the drug may produce delayed effects such as prolonged depression which may last for weeks or months. In some people LSD may precipitate schizophrenia, and there have been reports that LSD can cause damage to the chromosomes and to the foetus in the womb.

From the psychiatrist's point of view LSD can be of use in psychotherapy. It can enable psychiatrists to experience for themselves some of the feelings of a schizophrenic patient. It can be used for experimentally inducing psychoses which can then be studied in a more precise manner than those occurring naturally. This can aid in the development of drugs to counteract these psychoses.

Another hallucinogen is tetrahydrocannabinol, the principle constituent of cannabis. This is known by a number of names, for example, hashish, hemp, and marijuana. Many preparations of cannabis can be made from the hemp plant. Marijuana is a Mexican term for the chopped preparation of leaves and stems. It is usually smoked, as is hashish, which is in fact the only cannabis derivative that regularly produces hallucinogenic effects; hashish is roughly ten times as strong as marijuana. It contains nearly all the tetrahydrocannabinol in the plant. Hashish is commonly crumbled and mixed with tobacco to make 'reefers', which are smoked, and in this form is often referred to as 'pot' or 'grass'. In 1937 use of marijuana became illegal in the United States, but its use is becoming increasingly widespread. In 1964 there were 554 convictions for the use of cannabis in the United Kingdom, and by 1969 this figure had risen to 4683. Of course these figures are only a very rough index and probably represent a mere fraction of the actual use.

Tetrahydrocannabinol, like LSD, alters the level of two neurotransmitters in the brain. Unlike LSD, however, it does not stimulate throughout the body the 'fight-and-flight' systems, which alter the levels of chemicals (adrenaline, for example) in the blood.

After taking cannabis an individual experiences a drowsy sense of euphoria, during which considerations of time and space are forgotten, and a floating sensation, commonly termed 'being high'. During this stage the subject is more talkative. The euphoria is followed by a period in which perceptions are heightened and even changed. Thus in addition to colours becoming brighter, sounds more acute, and perfumes stronger, colours may be 'heard' and sound may be 'seen'. This 'psychedelic experience' has been the subject of a great deal of spurious intellectualizing.

The use of psychedelics has become fashionable, and a subculture has grown up centred round their use. There is talk of these drugs aiding artistic creation and improving one's appreciation of some sorts of music, but it is more likely that the effect of the drug is to give a false worth or significance to something that may, in reality, be artistically worthless; that is, to give increased subjectivity and diminish rational aesthetic response. In passing, it is interesting to note that the concept of psychedelic music is by no means a new one. The Russian composer Scriabin associated musical keys with colours, for instance, he visualized F major as 'the blood red of hell', and in 1910 composed his work *Prometheus* in which, in addition to using a large orchestra, piano, organ, and choir, he wrote a completely notated part for a 'colour organ'. The purpose of this was to express the musical sounds in terms of colour. Thus it would appear that in certain very creative individuals a 'psychedelic experience' may occur without recourse to any drug.

There is a vocal minority who wish to legalize cannabis so that it may be used socially as a pleasure-giving drug. To justify this they say that cannabis is safe and less harmful than alcohol. Although there is no evidence that cannabis is addictive or that it precipitates serious mental illness, it is possible that social factors may cause it to be a transition stage to the use of other more damaging and dangerous drugs. The claim that cannabis is less harmful than alcohol is difficult to substantiate by scientifically valid data since the data about cannabis have so far been drawn largely from population samples which differ ethnically and culturally from those of western civilizations which drink alcohol.

In a survey carried out in Brazil, India, Morocco, and Nigeria during the late 1950s and early 1960s it was found that 22.5 per cent of psychiatric hospital admissions were patients suffering from mental disturbances following self-administration of cannabis. In 1968 the percentage of the first admissions to psychiatric hospitals in Dublin that were suffering from alcoholism was twenty-five per cent (male) and five per cent (female). In terms of the damage to society caused by cannabis and alcohol the available data shows little difference between the two drugs. In 1965 half of those who committed crimes in three West African countries carried them out while under the influence of cannabis. A quarter of these crimes were of a sexual nature. An analysis of British ex-prisoners in 1966 revealed that half were heavy alcohol drinkers and of these eighty-nine per cent considered that alcohol played some part in causing them to commit their last crime.

Evidence from V.D. clinics in the U.S.A., Great Britain, and Morocco suggests that promiscuity is high among cannabis users. There is also evidence that there is a greater risk of the disruption of marital relationships among cannabis users.

It is well established that alcoholism causes loss of working time and diminished efficiency and intellectual performance, and there is also evidence that this is true of cannabis use. In 1944 the Mayor's Committee on Marijuana found that marijuana users had a poor and irregular work record. A similar conclusion was reached by Wilson and Linken in 1968, who showed that use of cannabis impaired the intellectual performance of students.

Thus the evidence, albeit sketchy, does not really bear out the claims that cannabis is harmless. It is clear that it produces antisocial behaviour in a proportion of its users and is likely to impair intellectual performance. In any case, when one surveys the ravages caused by alcohol abuse one should think very carefully before advocating the introduction of another social drug whose advantages over alcohol as regards social acceptibility are by no means proven, and whose dangers are, as yet, not fully understood.

Cannabis has been used therapeutically for the treatment of depression but it is incapable of producing complete or lasting remission. It has also been used in the treatment of narcotic withdrawal symptoms but has now been largely superseded by more specific and effective drugs.

Simpler substances that effect the brain

In addition to the complicated organic molecules (that is, chemicals built up primarily of carbon and hydrogen) which have been discussed so far, there are a number of very simple substances, such as metals and their salts, which are known

to affect the brain. Some have been found useful as therapeutic agents in psychiatry.

Lithium salts are being used increasingly for the control
of manic depressive illness. Lithium is the lightest metal
known and resembles both sodium and magnesium in its
chemical properties. However, whereas sodium and magnesium are essential constituents of human cells, lithium
is present only in traces. Lithium was first used as a cure
for gout (because its salt with uric acid is soluble), but it
was only in 1949 that its psychoactive properties were fully
realized.

The whole problem of manic depressive illness and the
therapeutic mode of action of lithium is still a flourishing
area of research. Some think that lithium affects transmitters in the brain, but evidence is increasing for the idea
that lithium can alter the distribution of sodium ions in the
body. Sodium ions play a crucial part in the transmission of
the nervous impulses.

A nerve impulse is a travelling wave of chemical and
physical events which involve, in particular, the nerve membrane. The energy for the impulse is provided locally along
the course of the nerve fibre and not by the stimulus (at the
synapse) which sets the impulse going. An impulse travels
along the nerve when sodium ions travel through the membrane into the nerve and potassium ions travel through the
membrane and out of the nerve; this results in a wave of
depolarization. This reverses the situation that is found in
the resting nerve, where sodium ions are in a higher concentration outside than inside and potassium ions are in a
higher concentration inside than outside. Thus before the
nerve can conduct another impulse this resting situation
must be restored. This is done by 'pumping' the sodium
ions back to the outside again. This sodium pump is an
enzymic mechanism that requires chemical energy. There is
now experimental evidence that lithium can alter the workings of the sodium pump. This is important because it has
also been demonstrated in patients that the distribution of
sodium in the body during mania is different from that in
depression.

Whereas lithium is a relatively recent addition to therapeutic weaponry, a number of other metals have been em-
ployed medicinally for thousands of years. An example of
such a metal is silver, although it is not used nowadays. The
reasons for its use were more astrological than pharmacological. The ancients believed that a relationship existed
between silver and the moon and that insane individuals
were under the influence of the moon goddess Luna (hence
the term 'lunatic'). As a consequence silver and its salts
were used in the treatment of nervous disorders and even as
recently as the late nineteenth century silver nitrate was
used to treat epilepsy.

Mercury is another example of a metal that was used
widely in the past—for example, in the treatment of
syphilis—but whose use is steadily diminishing owing to the
appearance of non-mercurial antiseptics and antibiotics.
However, compounds of mercury are widely used indus-
trially for a number of purposes (such as in some paints and
as fungicides) and thus the toxic effects of mercury are still
of considerable importance. In cases of mercury poisoning
the central nervous system is especially involved. In particular, prolonged exposure to organic compounds of mercury can have very grave consequences, including
behavioural changes, irritability, insomnia, shaking and
tremor, loss of balance, constriction of the visual field, and
sometimes severe mental illness. One of the most horrifying
illustrations of the effects of mercury poisoning is provided
by the tragedy at Minnemata in Japan, where mercury
pollution in the sea resulted in the whole population of the
area becoming afflicted with these symptoms and a number
of very severely mentally handicapped children being
born.

Lead, like mercury, is more important for its toxic effects
than for its therapeutic properties—indeed the toxic effects
of lead were first observed by Hippocrates in the second
century B.C. Although the gradual disappearance of lead
plumbing and the decline in the use of white lead in paints
has reduced two of the main risks of lead poisoning, there
is still the risk of lead pollution in the air from automobile

exhausts because tetraethyl and tetramethyl lead are used as anti-knock additives to petrol.

In common with mercury, the high lipid (fat) solubility of organic compounds of lead results in it gaining access to nervous tissue in significant quantities. Lead is excreted to a very limited extent, and if the daily intake is more than 0.6 milligrams, lead accumulates in the body. The most serious manifestations of lead poisoning are in the central nervous system, although some of the other symptoms such as severe abdominal pain and muscular weakness ('lead palsy') are also serious. Initially there is insomnia and disturbing dreams followed by loss of appetite, irritability, and anxiety. This is followed by loss of balance, exaggerated muscular movements, and confusion. Finally there may be delirium, visual disturbances, severe convulsions, and mania. In acute cases of lead poisoning the fatality rate is twenty-five per cent, and of the survivors approximately a fifth have paralysis and two-fifths have brain damage which may affect intelligence and behaviour.

The dangers of drugs

Throughout this chapter I have stressed the potential dangers of psychoactive drugs, probably at the expense of their undoubted value in medicine. Indeed, many experts in pharmacology are anxious about the present widespread over-use of these drugs. This over-use is not restricted to the abuse of narcotics and hallucinogens by certain sections of society, but is prevalent in society at large—as is witnessed by the huge consumption of barbiturates and the wide use of minor tranquillizers, to which I have already referred.

All these drugs act by blocking some particular part of the brain's activity, and no one can say (as yet) whether such actions will not also damage or lead to some destruction of the particular brain mechanism. It will be remembered from Chapter 9 that any neuronal damage is irreversible and irreparable. There is therefore a pressing need to study the effect of psychoactive drugs on the brain performance of those who use them over considerable periods of time.

Food and the brain

To conclude this chapter I must make a brief mention of the way in which the brain can be affected by our eating and drinking habits.

We have already seen how substances like the caffeine in coffee can affect mental performance, but there are also numerous examples of foods which are traditionally regarded (usually without any scientific foundation) as having a beneficial effect upon the brain—fish being the classic example. However, as was stressed in the preceding chapter, an adequate, well-balanced diet is a prerequisite for normal brain growth and function. It is far easier to point to substances which, when missing from the diet, cause serious brain malfunction, than to substances which, when added to a normal adequate diet, improve brain performance. Foods like fish are beneficial only because they are a good source of animal protein.

The vitamin content of food is extremely important to the brain since vitamins participate in virtually all the metabolic systems that provide energy and structural components for the nervous system. Deficiencies of vitamin B_6 can result in dementia and mental retardation, and a deficiency of another B vitamin, thiamine, has been implicated in the neurological changes that occur in Korsakoff's syndrome (see Chapter 8), infantile beri beri, and other diseases attacking the brain. The damaging effects of vitamin A deficiency in nervous tissue occur predominantly in the eye, with the result that vision can be permanently impaired. The importance of vitamin A for vision accounts for the belief that eating carrots is good for the eyes— carrots are a source of vitamin A.

Deficiencies of minerals and trace elements in the diet can also lead to severe mental disturbances. A lack of magnesium and calcium (required as activators of a number of important enzyme systems) can precipitate convulsions and mental confusion. A lack of iodine (required as a constituent of the thyroid hormones) causes the abnormality of brain development and activity known as 'cretinism'. In addition to being critical for the smooth functioning of the normal brain, a correctly controlled diet is important in the management of a number of mental illnesses. This is particularly true of the group of diseases caused by what are called 'inborn errors of metabolism'. These are hereditary illnesses due to a change in the body's genetic make-up which results in an important enzyme activity being absent. The most common example of this type of disease is 'phenylketonuria' which afflicts one in 10 000 live births.

In this country all babies are 'screened' for phenylketonuria by a simple blood test made soon after birth. The missing enzyme in the case of this disease is the one which converts the amino acid phenylalanine to another amino acid, tyrosine. This absence results in a build-up of phenylalanine itself and of its abnormal products. The reactions leading to the synthesis of several neurotransmitters including noradrenaline and 5-HT are also affected, so the brain is particularly vulnerable to this disease. The mental retardation caused by phenylketonuria is obvious when the child is a few months old. However, if a phenylalanine-free diet (avoiding ordinary milk and bread) is started during the first few weeks of life, the child will develop normally.

Since the time of Hippocrates attempts have been made to treat epilepsy by dietary control. Some claim that starvation reduces the frequency of fits, but obviously this is a rather unrealistic therapeutic measure. However, it is known that large meals may precipitate fits in epileptic children. A number of dietary restrictions such as reducing the intake of animal protein, sodium, and water have been suggested, but there is no scientific evidence that they are effective.

However, scientifically controlled studies have shown that certain dietary constituents can precipitate headaches in migraine sufferers. Citrus fruits, chocolates, wines and spirits, and cheese have been particularly implicated, and elimination of these items from the diet significantly reduces the frequency of migraine attacks. Recently it has been discovered that both cocoa beans and cheese contain a substance called 2-phenylethylamine, and it is thought that there is a connection between this common ingredient and migraine attacks. It may be possible to manufacture cheese which does not contain 2-phenylethylamine.

It may now be possible to treat some types of mental disorder by dietary control rather than by the administration of drugs. Researchers at the Massachusetts Institute of Technology have recently discovered that certain diets, when administered to rats, alter the level of the brain neurotransmitter 5-HT. It seems possible that the results obtained with rats will also apply to man. A lack of 5-HT in humans is associated with depression, thus it may be possible to treat this condition with an increased level of 5-HT provided by a suitable diet. In the Massachusetts experiments it was discovered that, although the effect of insulin is to lower the over-all amino acid level in the blood, the amount of the amino acid tryptophan is increased. And tryptophan happens to be the amino acid from which 5-HT is synthesized. Thus increasing the level of tryptophan in the blood increases the rate of synthesis of 5-HT.

Diets rich in carbohydrates stimulate insulin secretion; the researchers therefore fed their rats on high-carbohydrate diets to see if the brain 5-HT levels were increased. They were. However, when the diet was supplemented with protein there was no such effect. This paradox was resolved by the discovery that the amino acids in the blood derived from the high protein intake competed with the tryptophan for the carrier mechanism which transports amino acids to the brain. Thus an increase in 5-HT is achieved only with a diet *high* in carbohydrate but *low* in protein. And presumably this is the type of diet that would be required in the control of depressive illnesses.

5-hydroxtryptamine proves to be an interesting neurotransmitter in yet another respect. A reduced 5-HT level is known to promote sexual activity. And so perhaps a meal *high* in protein but *low* in carbohydrate may be an aphrodisiac, by reducing the 5-HT levels in the brain.

Should we all (and perhaps especially the 'slimmers' amongst us) be more interested in and informed about the effect our diet has upon our brains? The prospect of extending the present lines of research gives rise to some interesting speculations. Can a meal of high protein but low carbohydrate content be an aphrodisiac? Can there be a dietary control for certain mental illnesses? The initial evidence seems encouraging.

11

Education: how to make the best use of your brain

I have made a number of references to physiological mechanisms related to the maturing of the brain during the early months of life and to their possible importance for infant guidance and training in the early stages of education. The study of the brain from this point of view should be of great interest to all those concerned with the maturation and education of children.

The number of facts that can be stored in the brain (and the rate at which they can be assimilated) varies greatly from one brain to another, and some people discover—probably quite by accident—a method of processing the incoming information which is more effective than that used by others. These people are likely to excel in examinations, and may in extreme cases be said to have photographic memory. But a very important question for education is, how much factual information should be stored in the brain? Is it best to try and turn ourselves into 'walking encyclopaedias'?—or is it possible that the brain resources might be put to some more advantageous use?

The infant

As the development of the brain seems to depend very much on repetitions it seems that the infant's first need is to be guided to take a pleasure and interest in exploring the environment, in order that he or she may develop a desire to learn and joy in learning. The encouragement of behaviour-patterns is a challenge, and the natural maturation of behaviour is closely concerned with copying the behaviour of others—brothers and sisters and the adults who look after the child.

Indoctrination in early life

Some people nowadays are so afraid of becoming involved in what they call 'indoctrination' of the young that they think it best to leave the infant to develop in his own way and to learn entirely by his own experience. From the physiological standpoint, this is a ridiculous attitude to adopt in caring for a child and it is probably also a harmful attitude in later life. The intelligent adult can do much to smooth the way of the child exploring the environment so that the urge to learn becomes more of a pleasure and less of a frustration. This early help by a devoted adult is so vital to a child's happy development that even misguided or rigid indoctrination seems to be better than leaving the child to 'mess about' without any guidance.

This is, of course, a difficult matter. On the one hand, the processes of advancement and civilization have depended on the formation of powerful nations, religions, sects, and tribes which have shown great enthusiasm for indoctrination. But, on the other hand, a dictatorial regime has often debased the best in human behaviour. But it seems to me most desirable that the young child should not be distracted from developing his brain skills in the very early years by having to make decisions about the simple problems of behaviour, and that the best environment at this time of life is one of kindly conformity.

Another physiological need for the very young child is a friendly relationship with an adult to whom he can talk, for he requires this practice in the early stages of the processes of thinking. As busy parents are often unable to provide this need, it may well be that alternative methods should be provided by the community.

The development of the brain: Language skills

I have already expressed the view (p. 17) that musical genius can develop only in one who has been exposed to music almost from the day of his birth, since only in this way can the hearing mechanism in an infant's brain evolve sufficiently during maturation for the child to develop his potential in this field later. If this hypothesis is correct, then we should try to ensure that the language territory of the brain is actively developed during infancy, so that it may acquire the structural capacity to develop skills at a later age without difficulty.

The area of brain used specially for language skills was described in Chapter 5 (p. 57). The build-up of this area depends on information being fed in from four main directions as follows.

1 and 2. *Hearing* and *vision* are the first to be used, and these are led in from the temporal and occipital lobes respectively; talking to an infant with a display of affection will ensure that the maturation of both these regions is adequate. A deaf infant is at a tremendous disadvantage in this respect.

3. Actively *speaking* or trying to speak is the next important input or feed-back to the language territory, so that the more the infant is encouraged to speak or make a noise, the better.

4. The amazing development of *hand-skills* is perhaps the most unique feature of the human brain, and it seems to me to be absolutely crucial that this enormous contribution to the language territory should be cultivated at the earliest possible age, and the question to consider is just how this can be achieved.

My suggestion is that, between the ages of two and three, the child should be encouraged to associate symbols with objects seen or spoken about, and that small children should become accustomed to seeing adults draw symbols in relation to their everyday life; symbols could be extensively introduced into television broadcasts for small children. The simplest useful symbol is, of course, a letter, such as d for dog, and as soon as a child can hold a pencil he should play games that involve drawing such symbols, by means of a stencil if necessary. These games are not designed to enable the three-year-old to read, but simply to encourage a very important part of the brain's language territory to mature properly for future use. I am told that the reported incidence of illiteracy in Russia is so low that no one believes the figures. The teaching in modern Russian schools is based largely on the teaching of Pavlov, one of the world's greatest neuro-physiologists, who was a believer in this type of conditioning.

Other skills

Language skills must always have first priority in education, for through these the main capacity and potential for learning in all its more complex aspects can develop. However, as useful learning of the academic variety can take place probably for only two or three hours a day, it is just as important to encourage many other skills in relation not only to the hands but also to the whole field of the auditory, visual, and athletic pursuits.

As has been explained in previous chapters, the consolidation of memories for learning purposes requires frequent 'periods of no learning' in order to allow what has been fed in to consolidate itself. This occurs especially during the hours of sleep, but a period of repetitive manual, sporting, constructive, or musical work may be equally useful in allowing the more language-orientated learning to consolidate.

Thus it seems best to encourage all potential skills, in order to avoid undue pressure on any one facet of development. Although there is plenty of good evidence to support the hypothesis that hand-produced symbols related to objects should be used to develop the language area of the brain, there are no doubt other effective ways of supplying this need, and the adoption of several parallel approaches to the development of this area probably constitute the best solution.

It seems very strange to me that our society tends to separate manual workers from those who occupy themselves with verbal skills and thoughts for, from the physiological point of view, the hand-skills are just as important and unique in man as are his language developments. Perhaps the best solution would be to expect all those whose education tends towards the academic to spend more of their period of study working on manual or other routine tasks (as students have to do in China). Such a system should prove beneficial to the students' physiological and mental development and performance, besides providing assistance to society as a whole.

Higher education

I hope that, as a former teacher, I may be allowed to comment on what seem to me to be some weaknesses in our present arrangements for higher education.

The number of young people who qualify for this supposed privilege is now very great, and it seems to me that as the line of least resistance they tend to drift into what I have often called the 'tunnel' of higher studies, without having much idea of what to expect at the other end. While in this tunnel, they become relatively isolated from the rest of the community, and from the point of view of the brain I think that this arrangement can suit only a minority of those concerned. It would be much better for many of these young students if they first became occupied with some manual task or trade within the community as a whole, and later developed their education as a part-time 'hobby' or, as many students already do, returned to academic studies after a year spent working in the community in one way or another. This would provide a more interesting life for most young people, and I think they would look back on the arrangement with satisfaction. After all, one cannot expect the brain to absorb new information for more than a small part of each day, so that many university students may find their lives boring and unproductive when compared with the much more varied life in the community that I am suggesting.

There seems to be a curious built-in vested interest to prolong the duration of higher education for any one degree or profession. The common idea is that the longer the course, the higher the salary should be. There must be few degree or training courses which can stand up to critical assessment in this regard. After all, there can be no such thing as a 'finished product' for teaching or nursing, and no possibility of turning out a know-all for the medical or legal professions. Least of all can there be a completed training for the artist or the student of social sciences. How much more sensible it would be if all higher training was reduced by one-third or more, and if the further necessary studies were made on a part-time basis while actually engaged in practical work of some kind. Indeed, it is doubtful whether some of the present university training programmes should ever have been constructed as full-time courses at all.

Using your brain for pleasure and contentment

I would advise the person who sees little aim in life to consider the advantages and pleasures of developing his own brain. He will soon discover that the acquisition of exceptional knowledge or skills can give much satisfaction, and the resulting contentment can well be sufficient to last a lifetime.

For some fortunate people, their employment or profession can be the vehicle for exercising their brains, but for others their occupation must, of necessity, be dull and repetitive. However, as I have explained in this book, new knowledge is easily consolidated by the brain during hours of repetitive drudgery, without any effort by the individual concerned, so none of us have any excuse for not keeping our brains active.

We must always remember that the brain can only fulfil its potential when supported by good bodily health. Its complex mechanism cannot function well when strained by fatigue or over-stimulated by drugs of any kind. Correct care and use of your brain is the key to a stimulating existence and ultimate contentment. Look after your brain.

Further reading

N. CALDER. *The mind of man*. B.B.C. Publications (1970).

S. DIMOND. *The double brain*. Churchill Livingstone, London (1972).

J. C. ECCLES. *The understanding of the brain*. McGraw–Hill, New York (1972).

H. CHANDLER ELLIOTT. *The shape of intelligence*. Allen and Unwin, London (1970).

R. L. GREGORY. *Eye and brain*. McGraw–Hill, New York (1966).

A. R. LURIA. *The working brain*. Penguin Books, Harmondsworth (1973).

R. MARK. *Memory and nerve cell connections*. Clarendon Press, Oxford (1974).

P. NATHAN. *The nervous system*. Penguin Books, Harmondsworth (1969).

S. ROSE. *The conscious brain*. Weidenfeld and Nicolson, London (1973).

W. RITCHIE RUSSELL. *The traumatic amnesias*. Oxford University Press (1971).

W. RITCHIE RUSSELL. *Brain, memory, learning*. Clarendon Press, Oxford (1959).

J. R. SMYTHIES. *Brain mechanisms and behaviour*. Blackwell, Oxford and Edinburgh (1970).

J. Z. YOUNG. *An introduction to the study of man*. Oxford University Press (1971).

Glossary

acetylcholine: one of the neurotransmitters.
adversive reactions: rare types of fit in which disease or injury of one cerebral hemisphere leads to twisting movements of body and eyes in the opposite direction.
alexia: inability to read.
amnesia: loss of memory.
amino acid: one of the 20 or so 'building-blocks' which make up proteins.
aphasia: inability to speak due to disease or injury of the language mechanisms in the brain.
axon: the single fibre by which a nerve cell activates other nerve cells.

biogenic amine: class of organic substance which acts as a transmitter between neurones.

central nervous system: the brain and spinal-cord.
chemical transmitter (neurotransmitter): a chemical which carries information across the synaptic gap.
clonic: repeated motor jerks of the body or limbs.
cortex: the blanket of nerve cells covering all parts of the cerebral hemispheres.

dendrites: the fibres by which a nerve cell is activated by other nerve cells—there are usually large numbers for each cell.
DNA, deoxyribonucleic acid: polymeric molecule which makes up the hereditary material of genes and chromosomes in the nuclei of cells.
dopamine: a biogenic amine from which noradrenaline can be synthesized in the body; it is believed also to have its own function in brain action. A reduced content is a feature of Parkinson's disease.
dominant cerebral hemisphere: the side of the brain (the left side

in most people) in which the processing of language functions takes place.

enzyme: a protein controlling chemical reactions in the body.

focal fit: a fit caused by injury or disease of the cortex concerned with a special function (vision, movement, smell, hearing, feeling etc.).

frontal lobes: in man these most forward areas of the brain are much larger than in other species and give him his greater potential.

functional disease: a disability for which no organic basis is found and for which there is evidence that psychological processes are the cause.

glia: cells in the brain which support and nourish the neurones.

grand mal: major epilepsy.

grey matter: the blanket of nerve cells that cover the cerebral hemispheres which is visible in a cross-section of the brain as a grey layer.

hippocampus: large brain structure deep in each temporal lobe—a part of the limbic system.

hysteria: a functional disorder causing what seems to be a severe disability, but which is psychologically produced and which, if recognized, can be cured by persuasion.

hypothalamus: situated at the back of the brain; the hypothalamus is associated with the limbic system.

inhibition: an important part of the brain activity, by which activity of nerve cells is blocked.

lesion: a term used to indicate a disordered part of the brain in the anatomical sense—for example, a 'frontal lesion'. This location is often the first step in diagnosis.

limbic system: interconnected parts of the brain which lie deep within each cerebral hemisphere. These seem to provide several vital functions in the correlation of various aspects of brain activity.

metabolism: the chemical processes whereby a living thing is maintained and by which energy derived from the breakdown of foodstuffs is made available for various forms of work.

minor hemisphere: the cerebral hemisphere (usually the right) which is not the dominant hemisphere.

motor: concerned with the control of movement.

myelin: a fatty substance which is the main constituent of the sheath or tube which envelops each nerve fibre.

nasal visual field: for the right eye, this is the left half of the visual field when looking ahead. For the left eye this is the right half of the field.

neuromata: small nerve fibres which grow at the ends of nerves exposed by amputation.

neurone: a cell specially adapted for the carrying of nerve impulses.

noradrenaline: a biogenic amine (also a hormone). It occurs chiefly in the 'lower' parts of the brain and acts as an excitatory transmitter.

occipital lobes: the back (posterior) part of the cerebral hemispheres, in one part of which visual information from the eyes arrives in the hemispheres.

optic radiation: a large nerve tract. There is one in each hemisphere which conveys visual information from the optic nerves through the brain to the occipital lobes.

parietal lobes: the mid-region of the cerebral hemispheres between frontal and occipital lobes.

petit mal: minor variety of epilepsy.

pituitary: gland situated at the back of the head. It secretes a chemical into the blood which causes the liberation of hormones, thus stimulating the body's activities.

post-traumatic amnesia: the time-interval between a concussive blow to the head and the subsequent return to full consciousness— this corresponds to the period for which there is subsequently no memory of events.

proteins: large molecules used in the body for many functions including building tissues. They are made up of amino acids.

psychoactive: acting on the brain.

psychosomatic: a bodily effect caused by psychological processes.

reticular formation: a slender but powerful pathway to all parts of the brain and the spinal cord originating in the brain-stem. It controls many basic bodily functions.

retrograde amnesia: after full recovery from concussive head injury there is usually amnesia for events that occurred just before the injury. This term is used in referring to the pre-injury memory gap, especially with respect to its duration.

RNA, ribonucleic acid: information molecule found in all living cells. Acts as an intermediary between DNA and protein synthesis.

senile dementia: complete mental failure caused by the severe varieties of degeneration that may occur in old age.

sense organs: organs such as the eye, nose, ear and muscles from which information is led into the central nervous system.

stimulus: some physical process (for example, an electric shock) which activates nerve fibres. The word is also used to describe the effect of a naturally occurring nerve impulse.

synapse: the point of contact through which the axon of one cell transmits into the dendrites or cell surface of another nerve cell.

synaptic cleft: the minute gap in the synapse across which an impulse passes from cell to cell by a chemical process—via a neurotransmitter.

temporal lobes: these lobes of the cerebral hemispheres lie below the parietal lobes and between the frontal and occipital lobes; one in each hemisphere.

temporal visual field: this term is used for the right half of the visual field when looking ahead with the right eye. For the left eye this is the left half of the field.

thalamus: vital masses of nerve cells which lie deep in the middle of each cerebral hemisphere.

transient amnesia: a severe disturbance of memory which lasts for a limited period, perhaps a few minutes or a few hours, before the subject recovers.

traumatic dementia: gross and permanent failure of mental capacity caused by extensive areas of brain destruction resulting from severe head and brain injury.

uric acid: crystals only slightly soluble in water, which cause gout and kidney stones when they come out of solution. Formed in the liver, it then circulates in the blood until excreted.

visual cortex: the areas of the brain in each occipital lobe which receive information from the eyes via the optic nerves and optic radiations.

visual field: on looking straight ahead it is normally possible to see objects to right or left, above or below the line of gaze throughout a range of about 90° in each eye, that is, 180° in all. This is the field of vision.

white matter: in a cross-section of a cerebral hemisphere this is the whitest, inner part, which consists of nerve fibres conveying impulses from one part of the central nervous system to another.

Index